THE
SEX
DIARIES

THE
SEX
DIARIES

Why Women Go Off Sex and Other Bedroom Battles

BETTINA ARNDT

MELBOURNE
UNIVERSITY
PRESS

MELBOURNE UNIVERSITY PRESS
An imprint of Melbourne University Publishing Limited
187 Grattan Street, Carlton, Victoria 3053, Australia
mup-info@unimelb.edu.au
www.mup.com.au

First published 2009
Text © Bettina Arndt, 2009
Design and typography © Melbourne University Publishing Limited, 2009

Designed by Nada Backovic and Alice Graphics
Typeset by Megan Ellis
Printed in Australia by Griffin Press

National Library of Australia Cataloguing-in-Publication entry:

Arndt, Bettina, 1949–
  The sex diaries: why women go off sex and other bedroom battles /
  Bettina Arndt.
  9780522855555 (pbk.)

  Includes index.
  Bibliography.

  Sex customs—Australia. Sexual ethics—Australia. Men—Australia—
  Sexual behaviour. Women—Australia—Sexual behaviour. Interpersonal
  relationships.

306.7

Contents

Acknowledgements

To my wonderful diarists, my heartfelt thanks for having the courage to share with me the most intimate details of your daily lives. You were all so amazing, writing with such honesty and openness about your feelings and letting me in on so many of your secrets. I loved being part of your lives for the months you were all writing for me, talking to many of you on the phone and even meeting up with a few of you. Every morning I would rush to my email to see what had happened the night before, knowing there would always be someone who stayed up until the wee small hours to write to me or crept out of bed first thing in the morning to fill me in on what was happening. It was particularly exciting to see so many couples begin to talk to each other more openly and watch some of the anger and tension disappear. Many of you have told me that you gained from the experience—which is really exciting. But through your willingness to share your stories, many others may learn to handle these delicate negotiations just that much more easily.

There were many people who helped make this book happen. Michael Frankel, Morris Averill and Oliver Freeman were invaluable in helping me find the right publisher—Melbourne University Press. And the very professional team at MUP has made this book a remarkably easy process. It was so heartening to have the indefatigable Louise Adler throwing her support behind the book, while my publisher, Elisa Berg, nursed the project through to its fruition, offering endless sound advice and professional support. Thanks must also go to others in the MUP team: Cinzia

Cavallaro, Jacqui Gray, Terri King and Dina Kluska. The ever-patient Paul Smitz dealt with the onerous tasks of correcting my punctuation and picking up glitches in my sometimes slapdash grammar and idiosyncratic expression.

My research assistant, Carrie Lumby, was a great help in helping me prepare for the project, setting up the database and computer system required to coordinate the vast quantities of diary material that flooded in each day. She was a delight to work with, endlessly cheerful, smart, insightful and as fascinated by the intricacies of sexual relations as I am—the perfect assistant for this very special project.

Many experts devoted valuable time to helping me get things right, like Juliet Richters from the University of New South Wales, Gemma O'Brien from the University of New England and the ever-generous Rosie King, who made numerous corrections and offered enthusiastic support for the project.

Then there were my extraordinary friends. Some were even willing to do diaries for me and participated in the trial run that led to the final project. It's bad enough writing about such things for a total stranger, but for my friends to do it was a rare act of daring and kindness. I am most grateful. There were many others, like my dear friend Judy Black and my surrogate mother, Enid Barnes, who were both always there, making the right encouraging noises. I was especially lucky to have as my sounding board the witty, razor-sharp Kate Legge, a successful fellow author who was the perfect person to critique early drafts and offer solace in dark moments. And it was her husband, Greg Hywood—one of the most emotionally intelligent men I know—who came up with the idea of a book exploring the gender gap over the sex supply.

For my children, it wasn't easy. They put up with their distracted mother brooding over her all-consuming project and suffered through embarrassing teasing from their friends, who delighted in asking her to tell all. My younger son, Cameron, had the worst of it, as the only child still living at home. But he dealt with even the most blush-inducing revelations at the Arndt dinner table with his usual charm and good humour. Thanks must also go to very special men in my life, past and present, who have taught me what it is all about.

1

Fifty Thrusts and Don't Jiggle My Book

There is a wonderful scene in the movie *Annie Hall* in which the camera switches between Woody Allen in his psychiatrist's office and his lover, Diane Keaton, in hers. They are each asked how often they have sex.

'Hardly ever', Allen says plaintively. 'Maybe three times a week.'

'Constantly', Keaton groans. 'I'd say three times a week.'

That's the scene that everyone remembers even thirty years after the movie was released. It touches on a great truth about relationships—that after the first lusty years are over, most men want more sex than their female partners. Of course, it's not always the case. There are passionate women who never lose interest and some men who do. But if we walked through the streets of Australia asking who's not getting enough, there'd be ever so many more male hands than female hands waving in the air.

In 2006, the BBC reported: 'A woman's sex drive begins to plummet once she is in a secure relationship. Researchers from Germany found four years into a relationship, less than half of 30-year-old women wanted regular sex'.[1] There's still a steady stream of such stories, news reports suggesting that women go off sex. All over the world, researchers are scurrying around to try to pin down the cause. Is it to do with hormones, or brain chemistry? Is it part of an evolutionary legacy? What's the role of the psyche in all of this? But there's no doubt it happens, and everyone knows it. It has entered our marital folklore and become an accepted part of our personal dynamics. Hang around a pub for long enough and you'll hear the jokes about the fallout—the sexually starved men. Like the story of the cow from Woy Woy.

The only cow in a small town in Victoria stopped giving milk. Eventually the townspeople found a replacement cow in Woy Woy, New South Wales, which proved a gem. It produced lots of milk and everybody was very happy. They decided to breed with it, so they bought a bull and put it in the pasture with their beloved cow. However, whenever the bull came close, the cow would move away. The people were very upset and asked the local vet what to do.

'Whenever the bull approaches our cow, she moves away', they said. 'If he approaches from the back, she moves forward. When he approaches her from the front, she backs off.'

The veterinarian thought for a moment and asked, 'Did you buy this cow in Woy Woy?' The people were dumbfounded since they hadn't mentioned where they had bought the cow. 'You are truly a wise vet', they said. 'How did you know we got the cow in Woy Woy?' The veterinarian replied, with a distant look in his eyes, 'My wife is from Woy Woy'.

I've spent much of the last thirty-five years listening to stories about wives from Woy Woy. From the time I started working as a sex therapist back in the early 1970s, people have been talking to me about their sex lives. What I hear about most is the business of negotiating the sex supply. How do couples deal with the strain of the man wishing and hoping while all she longs for is the bliss of uninterrupted sleep? It's a night-time drama being played out in bedrooms everywhere, the source of great tension and unhappiness.

But this drama is usually a silent movie, with couples rarely talking about the subtle negotiation that goes on between them. His calculations: 'What if I …? Will she then …?' Her tactics: dropping her book as he appears at the bedroom door and feigning sleep; staying up late in the hope that he'll doze off. Tensions. Resentment. Guilt. And then there are the rare couples who magically maintain mutual lust for each other.

That's what this book is all about. Through radio interviews and magazine articles, I recruited ninety-eight couples to spend six to nine months keeping diaries for me, writing about their daily negotiations over sex.[2] They are couples of all ages, from 20-year-old students to people in their seventies who have been married over forty years—young couples at the start of their relationships; pregnant women; couples caught up in the exhaustion of young families; women who want more sex than their husbands and women who'd live happily without it; older couples dealing with health issues like prostate surgery and arthritis. Some wrote every day for months—one man ended up providing over seventy pages of details of his love-life—while others provided only brief weekly summaries. As I expected, the cow from Woy Woy took centre stage.

Women know their loss of sexual drive is a huge issue in their relationships. Many write saying they can't bear what it is doing to their men. They understand their resentment but they feel they can't help it; they just rarely want sex any more. 'I hate it that I don't have a sex drive like before. I would do anything … well almost anything', writes Nadia (aged forty-one) from Sydney.

Listen to Judy. 'If there's an OFF switch in the female body, mine was turned many years ago', writes the fifty-eight year old from Bathurst, New South Wales, explaining that sex has been the single most divisive issue in her 27-year marriage. She's had enough: 'I have found that my already low libido has pretty much disintegrated and sexual interest is right up there with algebra, housework and trying on bras!'

Her husband has a strong drive and used to want sex twice a day, but hers has always been low: 'I'm actually quite inhibited, don't like experimenting and generally find sex and everything that goes with it a big yawn. If there was a drug that turned women on, I would not be the slightest bit interested'. They have fought about sex for years and she's finally persuaded him to back off a little. Now they are down to having it a few times a week. 'I'd still rather read a book', she says, adding:

> I just feel bloody guilty. I sense when he is feeling like sex, and I psych myself and prepare myself to cope. Shit, that sounds dreadful but it's the truth. I think having sex when you don't really want it is the most horrible thing. Once I would still respond, and even have orgasms despite not wanting it but now I don't have any response at all, so it feels horrible. Inside, I'm screaming for it to be over quickly, but outside I'm pretending … moving with him, grabbing his back, making him feel that I'm with him. But I'm not. I think he suspects; in fact, I'm sure he suspects, but it's a game we both play.

Judy knows how much it hurts him that she's not interested.

> The hardest thing is that he knows I don't enjoy it. It drives him to distraction. There is always a tension there, though it's never actually stopped him doing it! Must be dreadful for him. When he finishes, he's always got a kind of 'pissed off' vibe, and, believe me, I totally understand but gosh I wish I got the same kind of understanding for where I'm at, not the underlying unspoken accusation that there's something wrong with me.

She adds, sadly: 'It seems most partnerships are terribly out of sync. How nice to be in harmony with desire. Does it exist?'

Oh yes, it exists. 'I have no recollection of ever being refused sex', writes Rob, a very happy man from Perth, married for over forty-four years. What a treat it is to read this couple's diaries. His wife, Jenny, comes in for a cuddle at the breakfast table and undoes her dressing gown, exposing her breasts so he can kiss and nuzzle them. Often he comes into the shower with her. 'I rub his penis in my slippery hands which feels good for both of us', Jenny tells me. Her husband explains that Jenny's enjoyment of lovemaking has always been as fulfilling as his, and describes it as an integral part of their loving relationship. 'I am still moved by the beauty of her body, her breasts, which are still very beautiful to me, and I love seeing her vulva, imagining myself kissing her clitoris and seeing her lips swell in preparation for my penis to enter', says the passionate 65-year-old.

It has always amazed me to hear such stories of long-lasting passion. From the time that I first started talking about sex on television and radio, the couples who really love sex have reached out to me. I remember buying a ticket at an airport when a fifty-ish saleswoman looked left and right, leaned over to me and whispered, 'Isn't sex wonderful!' I have long known about the lusty couples who spend a remarkable amount of their lives between the sheets. They are the lucky ones. Yet they are rare and sadly outnumbered by the men and women who struggle, day after day, with the corrosive effect on their relationship of women's low libidos.

With my sex diaries, it was the men's stories that really set me back on my heels. It is so rare that men talk openly about such personal issues, but the diaries gave them permission to let loose. Every day I received page after page of eloquent, often immensely sad diary material, as men grasped the opportunity to talk about what quickly emerged as being a mighty emotional issue for them. Men might tell jokes about sexually deprived husbands, but talk to them privately and they aren't laughing—that was the most powerful message emerging from the many thousands of pages of personal communication in the diaries. Men aren't happy. Many feel duped, disappointed, in despair at finding themselves spending their lives begging for sex from their loved partners. They are stunned to find their needs so totally ignored. It often poured out in a howl of rage and disappointment.

Andrew from Queanbeyan, New South Wales, is forty-one years old, has been married for six years to Lorraine, and has two girls aged four and two. The couple started off having sex every day, sometimes twice a day, but sex has been on the decline ever since—now Andrew is lucky to have sex once every five to six months.

He's a very upset man:

> I am totally at a loss as to what to do. I do love her and I think she loves me but I cannot live like a monk. I have deliberately tried not to mention sex much at all but now I am so frustrated I don't know what to do. I am at breaking point. I cannot and will not continue on like this. I refuse to go through life begging.

He knows he's not alone. He simply can't understand how men ended up with such a dud deal:

> What makes women think that halfway through the game they can change the rules to suit themselves and expect the male to take it[?] If we started to abuse them or treat them badly, that … is totally unacceptable, but for them to do this to us is a part of life and acceptable. I JUST DO NOT GET IT!!!!!!! What about the male?????? The new world expects the male to be a provider, father, understanding husband, considerate and everything else. Well that is ok but if he does not get his needs met, who gives a shit?

'Would you like to change sex in any way?' was the question asked by US sex researcher Shere Hite of the 7000 men who responded to her survey. 'More, I just want more', came the overwhelming reply. 'We live in a sex economy that produces an ongoing pool of surplus male desire, a world that gives men precious little opportunity to feel desired, feel desirable and appreciated for our sexual natures', one man told Hite.[3]

Yet for men, this is usually a private misery. So many men writing to me report that they have never before told anyone about the sexual tension they experience. Like Nick, for example—a 53-year-old retired police officer from Melbourne. He tells me his sex life is non-existent. His erection problems are part of the story, but also his wife has no sex drive:

> I love my wife dearly and we have a fabulous marriage and care for each other very deeply. I still find my wife sexually attractive and would love to make love to her. I understand that we are getting older but I miss the affection and the closeness of making love to my wife. Over the past several years I have really suffered in silence to the point I could just sit down and cry. I mean, a male my age does not cry, nor does he speak about the problem.

How different is that from the way most women deal with it? Many of the women report amusing stories of sharing the issue with their friends, exchanging tips, offering each other solace for the business of dealing with grumpy husbands. Their tales are often very funny. I loved the woman who wrote to me complaining that her husband claimed his ability to get an erection would fade away if his cock wasn't continually exercised. 'This is a man who seriously spends too much time listening to the paranoid rantings of his trouser sage', she added wryly.

Judy offers funny reports from cappuccino sessions with her friends. She mentions one woman who has cancer: 'She said at a recent get-together that now she's growing her hair back and feeling a lot better she's realised that her husband has got used to going without sex and she's not about to remind him!' Another of Judy's friends, who has had no interest in sex for years, said that recently her husband wanted sex and she read her book while he was doing it. 'Can't quite get my head around that', Judy adds.

What is it with this reading business? US comedian Emo Philips once quipped, 'My girlfriend always giggles during sex—no matter what she's reading'. I'd always assumed it was just a joke, but then a friend of mine mentioned how a member of her book club had lain down conditions for sex with her husband —'You can have fifty thrusts but don't jiggle my book', she told him.

It may sound startling, but after so many years of sitting around with women, hearing stories about their sex lives, nothing would surprise me. I've certainly contributed to these conversations, shared in the general hilarity over the stories of how to get out of having sex. Like staging a fight last thing at night, knowing that then he won't approach you. Or pretending to be sick. Or being delighted when he gets a late-night business call so then you can feign sleep by the time he returns to bed. There was a time when I felt just the same, when I too announced I'd be happy never to have sex again. Female solidarity on this issue is so very comforting. It is only when you listen to men talking honestly about what it's like to be on the receiving end that you realise the impact of the contempt with which we treat them.

Back in the early 1960s, Betty Friedan wrote in *The Feminine Mystique* about 'the problem that has no name'—women's un-voiced frustrations with their housewifely role.[4] Women live unexamined lives, she said, talking about the strange stirring, vague sense of dissatisfaction and unvoiced yearning suffered by women in the middle of the twentieth century. By naming the problem, she encouraged women to say 'I want something more'. And we have been saying it, very loudly, ever since.

But now it is men who live unexamined lives. Men live day by day never publicly voicing their discontent, keeping their hidden yearnings to themselves. Their 'problem that has no name' is sexual frustration.

One reason it is so rarely discussed is that men experiencing sexual rejection feel ashamed. It is not the sort of thing they are likely to discuss with their mates or broadcast to the world. Songwriter Fred Small writes:

> Economic and political realities notwithstanding, most men do not perceive women as powerless, in part because women hold the power of rejection. I suspect that a man who whistles at women on the street actually perceives women as having more sexual power than he. We are trained from childhood to believe that real men get sex from women, that if we do not get sex from women, we are not men, we are nothing.[5]

It takes courage for men to admit to each other that they are not 'real men'. Gradually, my male diarists started to talk about the issue with other men. I received a steady trickle of letters from men reporting they had discovered that their friends were also on short rations. Sydney man Clive (aged forty-eight) had a long talk to his best mate, who reported he spent his life grovelling for sexual favours from his wife:

> This is a guy who is the salt of the earth, devoted husband and father, doesn't play around, works really hard and gives his family a good standard of living and I just shake my head. He is a martyr for his family but doesn't seem to be appreciated or given much in return.

Clive has three sons. He thinks about what their marriages will be like. Will they too spend their lives grovelling for sex?

> Unless some of us are prepared to speak out nothing will ever change. If we were to speak out in public (most of the people

I know are professional people and would be frankly too scared to speak out) we would most likely be ridiculed, accused of being deviates, sexual fiends, perverts, and most likely they would not understand why our wives would bother to still even live with us.

It is clearly very rare for men to speak out about the issue, but Nigel Marsh is an exception. He has written a very funny book about the year he spent taking stock after being fired from his job as an advertising executive. Yet what really struck a chord with readers of his bestselling *Fat, Forty and Fired* was the brief chapter he wrote about sex. In it, Marsh tells the story of a married friend—monogamous, loving, in good shape—who doesn't think it is right or fair that he should be made to feel bad about wanting sex. He decides he needs to ascertain first where sex ranked in his wife's priorities:

'Sweetheart, is sex as important to you, say, as a holiday away?' he started.

'No? Okay, how about a weekend away?' he continued.

'No? That's fine. A good meal?' he suggested.

This line of questioning continued until, as Marsh writes, 'he got into a serious debate with his wife about whether sex was something she looked forward to more or less than cleaning the oven. She eventually settled on an equal ranking'.[6]

Nigel Marsh dared to suggest that men, especially married men with kids, aren't so much pussy-whipped as pussy-neglected. And he was knocked over in the ensuing rush of responses. Seven hundred men wrote to him to say they were permanently sexually frustrated, that their wives never initiated sex. Instead, one said, they 'dispense' it. Many of the men believed their wives lived in a willing state of denial: 'In their hearts they know their husbands aren't satisfied with boring, grudgingly dispensed sex once every three weeks, but they'd rather not talk about it. Because then they might have to do something about it'. Do something? Oh yes, Marsh has a solution: 'Bonk more'.

It's not as crass as it sounds. In his sequel, *Observations of a Very Short Man*, Marsh bends over backwards to say all the right things, spelling out the very good reasons why women lose interest, describing the innumerable issues women tell him must be sorted out before they will want sex.[7] But he bravely goes on to suggest that women might just find that having more sex may actually help them fix those other issues.

Of course, the question arises as to what we mean by 'sex' and whether women would be keener to participate if there was more of the lovemaking many of them preferred, such as the gentle touch of a slow hand, soft lips and tongue, rather than the lusty rutting many men prefer: more hors d'oeuvres and less main course, perhaps. But whatever the menu, there are also women out there suggesting that we do it more often. Trawl through the chat sites on the internet and, amid the men and women complaining about their sex lives, there's always a scattering of posts from women doing things differently.

'Of all the things you do in your daily life to make your husband happy, to keep your household running—how many of them give you physical pleasure?' asks a woman on a mothering website. She goes on: 'Well, what if I told you that your husband couldn't begin to care less if you did any of those things, so long as you did the one task that does give you pleasure?' She suggests that women often overcompensate for their lack of sex drive by working hard at domestic chores, assuming their husband will notice their sacrifice and think, 'Gee, no wonder she doesn't want sex. Look how hard she works'. But that's not going to happen, she continues. 'They don't see how hard you work. All they see is you're not having sex with them.' The writer suggests that women put sex on the to-do list—not every day, but maybe once or twice a week: 'Shag a little more than the low-libido partner would like and a little less than the high-libido partner would prefer and I swear to you, your marriage will improve in huge ways'.

Hang on a moment. Isn't that suggesting that women just do it? That sometimes they should have sex when they are not in the mood? The very suggestion runs into a massive ideological roadblock. Women's right to say 'no' has been enshrined in our cultural history for nearly fifty years. It was one of the outstanding achievements of the women's movement to outlaw rape in marriage and teach women to resist unwanted advances. But it simply hasn't worked to have a couple's sex life hinge on the fragile, feeble female libido. The right to say 'no' needs to give way to saying 'yes' more often—provided both men and women end up enjoying the experience. The notion that it might be in women's best interests to stop rationing sex is sure to raise hackles, but this is an issue that deserves serious attention.

The case is best made by a passionate letter I received when I first asked for volunteers for the diaries. The writer, Sam, is a 54-year-old, twice-married man from Brisbane whose first marriage fell apart over battles about sex:

> As my first marriage unravelled, two marriage counsellors were engaged by my first wife and me. The second counsellor asked me to take a week to think about my sex issues and to try to put my feelings into words. As it turned out, I didn't need a week. As I pondered her request, the answer came to me like a revelation. If sex is mutual, when both people want it, that's wonderful. If one partner wants sex and the other doesn't but offers it as a gift, that too is pretty darned good. But my first wife regularly refused, complaining about my unreasonable demands. Sometimes she begrudgingly complied, which made me feel like a thief, as if I had stolen something that was not rightfully mine. My advances were unwarranted and unwanted,

and I felt the way she so often wanted me to feel, unwelcome. Sex was rarely mutual and almost never a gift. After twenty-five years of marriage I decided I deserved happiness. I divorced her. A few years later I remarried.

Rose, my second wife of seven years, has a demanding job as a manager. Nevertheless, she has never said 'no'. She has never used the headache defence, never been too tired. Always, she makes sex a gift if she is not in the mood herself. Often she finds herself enjoying the moment. She does this because she cares about me, about my feelings and my needs. In my case, I'm sure you can guess the outcomes. If I notice Rose is run down and tired, seldom will I reach for her, other than to give her a cuddle. If she is not well, I look after her, tuck her into bed and either read or veg out in front of the TV. On the other hand I am perfectly capable of springing a sexual ambush on her as she walks through the door at the end of a long day. I am far from the perfect husband, but I do love and care for her, not because I am a wonderful bloke, but because her so very obvious caring for me can lead to little else other than reciprocity.

I approach Rose for sex less frequently than I did my first [wife], but we have more and better sex. We are the most happy and relaxed couple you are likely to meet. A sexually frustrated man will reach for his wife at every opportunity, until she drives him away with her selfishness and emotional barbs. However, a man who knows his wife loves him and cares for him, who knows she will be there for him when he needs or wants her, becomes very relaxed about sex. It becomes easy for him to be considerate, and to care for his wife. A starving man thinks about little else other than his own need for food. A sexually frustrated man becomes fixated on sex. Unfortunately, the more demands he places on his wife, the more frequently he is likely to be met with refusal or made to feel like an unwelcome glutton. This becomes an emotional vortex, sucking both of them into despair and unhappiness.

All this applies to any part of our lives together instead of being restricted to sex. Rose dislikes being left alone but if I feel like going on a camping trip with my sons, she encourages me. She is an introvert, and dislikes being dropped into a room full of people not known to her, so most of the time I stay close to her under these circumstances. We try to see each other's needs and to meet them …

It all seems so simple. If you love someone, you care for them; their needs and wants are as important as … yours. Each of us is unique in the ways in which we show our caring, and all of us fail sometimes. But if your women readers took the lead from my dear wife, they might just find that their grumpy, disgruntled husbands become what they once were and could be again, wonderful blokes who loved and cared for them enough to want to spend the rest of their lives with them.

Sam does make it sound simple. But it seems extraordinary that sex is treated so differently from all the other ways in which a loving couple cater to each other's needs and desires. We are willing to go out of our way to do other things to please each other—cooking his favourite meal, sitting through repeat episodes of her beloved television show. Why, then, are we so ungenerous when it comes to 'making love', which should be the ultimate expression of that mutual caring? 'Love is as love does', said M Scott Peck in *The Road Less Travelled*.[8] Surely, maintaining sexual intimacy is one of the crucial tests of doing love.

So the sex diaries weren't just about bad news. Yes, some documented the terrible tension, anger and resentment that erupts when couples clash over sex. But there were also diaries brimming with intense erotic adventures, so very, very sexy to read—couples writing about the sexual joy they share together; so many pages bearing witness to their tenderness, their loving, their caring. There are many couples who are getting it right—very right. They have much to teach us all.

2

Shifting the Sprinkler and Other Green Square Days

It's a quiet summer evening. A dog barks in the distance, an occasional car moves over the tree-lined hilltops. A woman is having a shower, cheerfully soaping her full breasts and washing off her slim hips and shapely legs. She's in great shape for her early sixties, her taut body bearing witness to her regular work-outs at the gym.

She can hear her husband pottering around his workshop as she dries herself and rubs moisturiser into her smooth skin. She runs a comb through her bouncing, shoulder-length brown hair and then heads for her underwear drawer. Not the one with her sensible daily wear, cottontails and gym bras. This one is special—a drawer filled to the brim with red satin corsets, lacy suspenders, black-lace bustiers, the briefest of thongs, G-strings —a veritable treasure chest of bodily adornment. She makes her selection, wriggles into the tight white-lace corset and at-taches the sheer silky stockings to her delicate suspenders. Then, a final touch, his favourite red stilettos, before heading for the kitchen.

This is the start of what Michael calls his 'Underwear Parade'. Here, in this unassuming suburban house in the Adelaide Hills, the 68-year-old retired engineer is treated to a loin-stirring erotic spectacle. Every evening, his wife, Heather, totters around on her high heels, preparing dinner, offering Michael his evening drink, laying the table, doing a few chores. And he watches in delight as her oh-so-tiny garments struggle to curtain her ample breasts and grip her tight buttocks. 'It's an added bonus if she hangs out the clothes or shifts the sprinkler', he tells me.

It wasn't only the story of the underwear parade that convinced me to spend some time with this intriguing couple. They had another secret. In the first brief note I had received from Michael, he mentioned he had records, very accurate records, of the last quarter-century of their sexual activity.

Accurate records indeed. Michael has used year-in-a-page calendars, like the ones that used to be handed out by the local butcher or grocery shop. He has completed twenty-three of these, with many of the 365 tiny squares filled with a brightly coloured code. Green square? That's a touchdown—mutual orgasms— and there are plenty of those. But sometimes there'll be a green triangle, which means only one of them climaxed, usually Michael. (Heather admits she doesn't climax easily but always enjoys sex.) There are red squares for her periods; green lines for 'serious' cuddles; tiny hands for masturbation; even the occasional four interlinked circles—that's the Audi symbol, meaning they'd had it off in their car. Day after day, square after square, it's all there. Their entire sex life in all its glory.

Why would he do this? Well, it all started when they were going through a very sexy period. 'It was curiosity, really. I just wanted to monitor a really great sex life', says Michael. He's a tall, lean man, with a still handsome but craggy face and piercing blue eyes, and has clearly been the driving force in their long and remarkably sexually active marriage. Heather tells me she suspects the calendars were also designed to put pressure on her to keep up the pace. When Michael starts writing a diary for me, I receive regular messages from Heather saying that, what with grandparent duties and other distractions, their sex life isn't what it used to be—which she clearly worries is letting down the side.

Their yearly total was way down, averaging only once a week compared with two to three times when the diaries began, which is when the couple really started to get adventurous. It was a wedding anniversary that triggered things. Michael had planned it down to the last moment: the Rolls-Royce rolling up their drive, whisking them down to Adelaide for a gondola ride on the river, followed by a candlelit dinner at the Hilton, then off to their hotel room to be greeted by a couple Michael had organised for a sexual adventure. Clothes disappeared and they all piled onto the huge bed. 'Oh yes, we watched them and they obviously watched us. There was much frivolity and laughter', says Michael. 'It was very arousing', admits Heather, adding that 'the ultimate orgasm was enjoyed after they left'.

There were a few other swinging adventures, plenty of green square days. These became a regular Saturday night event when they took up ballroom dancing—the tango does it for them every time. 'We have done everything over the years to keep life interesting', says Michael. 'Nude photography, nude bathing, sex in public locations, naked romps with friends, a brief swinging period.' And now that the children have left home, underwear parades almost every night. Occasionally their adult children will pop in unexpectedly. 'There's a mad scramble to the bedroom to put something else on', laughs Heather.

When I tell women about the underwear parade, they are stunned: You're kidding—every night in stilettos? They interpret Heather's evening ritual as that of a woman pandering to a man's sexual appetite, and the idea rankles. Yet many of these women think nothing of preparing a three-course meal for their man or searching shopping centres for his favourite brand of cotton socks. Somehow, seduction has come to be seen as an anti-feminist act, a betrayal of equality quite different from other nurturing gestures.

It's assumed there's nothing in it for her. Yet, talking to Heather, it's clear it also lights her fire. 'It makes me feel good. If I don't bother and end up spending the evening in a tracksuit, it makes me feel a slob', she says. But it is not just about avoiding feeling slothful. Here's a woman who revels in seeing herself as sexual.

The funny thing is that she's rather a shy woman, reluctant initially to talk about her own experiences and refusing to write a diary. She trained as a librarian and that's how she appears at our first meeting: demure but very attractive, dressed in a neat bright-yellow shirt, pencil skirt, stockings and heels. Yet as we chat over the light lunch she has prepared—salad and delicious whiting fillets—I catch glimpses of her raunchy side. She clearly enjoys parading around her garden in her finery—'I don't care if the neighbours know'—and mentions the birthday cake she prepared for a male friend, which she presented decked out in one of her lacy numbers at his party surrounded by all their friends. She delights in the male gaze, and later, the couple reap the rewards.

There are other couples writing for me who are also determined to keep sexuality centrestage in their marriages. Instead of spending their evenings reading books or nodding off in front of the television, these folk are ducking off to the bedroom to heat the massage oil or light the candles. Like Tasmanian couple Bob and Jan, married for thirty-three years. They are in their fifties and partially retired, but both drive school buses at the crack of dawn. They are home by 8.30 a.m. and often pop back into bed for a bit of nooky.

Then there's Meg and Paul, from Brisbane. She's fifty-six, he's sixty-one and they have been married for thirty-five years. They had sex every single night of their marriage, sometimes twice and occasionally three times a night. Then, last year, when Paul hit sixty, he had surgery for prostate cancer. 'That curtailed us but has not stopped us', says Meg, who firmly believes that the more sex in a marriage, the better. Erections are finally returning and their sex life is slowly getting back on track. 'Sex is our favourite activity together. What better way to pass an evening?' she adds.

Rikki (aged forty-seven) and Ted (fifty-nine) live and work together on a mango farm in northern Queensland, far away from all their neighbours. It's the perfect setting for their evening relaxation, often spent naked or only partially clothed. 'We usually shower together in our outdoor bathroom and this helps stimulate our sex life', says Ted. After dinner they may start to watch a little TV but often the sex starts before the show is finished. They have sex six or seven times a week and on the days they miss out, they kiss and cuddle and touch constantly.

Esther Perel would be proud of them. Her intriguing book *Mating in Captivity* challenges couples to reconcile their erotic and domestic lives, to 'bring home the erotic', as she puts it. 'Nurturing eroticism in the home is an act of open defiance', she writes, explaining that our cultural penchant for equality and togetherness is smothering erotic desire. Desire is fuelled by unknowns, she says. 'If intimacy grows through repetition and familiarity, eroticism is numbed by repetition. It thrives on the mysterious, the novel and the unexpected … Too often, as couples settle into the comforts of love, they cease to fan the flame of desire.'[1]

The efforts of couples like Heather and Michael to fan those flames leave most of us gasping. Oh, it is true that even these two have had the odd bad year. Their pre-children period was a little lean. 'I was on the Pill, blew up like a balloon. Michael was too busy working', says Heather. Lean, too, were the years with tiny children. And there were troubled times, such as when Heather decided to study librarianship. Michael wasn't at all happy about that—he became distant, so she rebelled and in 1979 had a brief affair with her hairdresser. Fifteen years later she finally told Michael about it, and the fallout is evidenced in the calendar—months of no green squares, just little hands and lots of green triangles as she made strenuous efforts to console him. And there were no green squares for weeks after the fatal day she cut her hair short and he didn't like it. But these are mere blips in a 43-year history that throbs with desire.

'The brave and determined couples who maintain an erotic connection are, above all, the couples who value it. When they sense that desire is in crisis, they become industrious and make intentional, diligent attempts to resuscitate it', Perel proclaims, explaining that intentionality conveys value. 'When you plan for sex, you are affirming your erotic bond … Longing, waiting and yearning are fundamental elements of desire that can be generated with forethought, even in long-term relationships.'

But what if neither of you really cares about that bond? Is it a problem if both of you really prefer tucking in to chocolate mousse or reading a book? 'If I had a choice between reading a good book and having sex, the book wins', says Joan Sewell, author of *I'd Rather Eat Chocolate*, cheekily acknowledging that the adjective 'good' is really just her attempt to put a better face on things. Her husband, Kip, would have sex five or six times a week if he could have as much sex as he wanted, compared with her preferred once or twice a month. 'There are times I wish I were a lesbian', Sewell moans, describing the efforts she has made to deal with the incompatibility of their drives.[2]

Lesbian bed death—that's what they call it when two feeble female libidos get together and Eros quickly dies a painless death.[3] Many heterosexual women look at their lesbian sisters and envy them, suggests Sandra Tsing Loh, writing on women's libido for

Lesbian Bed Death

Does 'lesbian bed death' really exist?

The notion that gay women who settle down together eventually succumb to a sexless love-life has been the subject of intense debate on gay websites across the world. Yet the evidence is clear. Lesbian couples do have less sex than other couples, such as heterosexuals or gay men. 'After two years together, lesbians have sex less frequently than married heterosexual couples do after ten years', reports Janet Lever, who compared responses to a survey in a gay and lesbian news magazine, *The Advocate*, with national data on heterosexuals.[4]

Lever's results echo Philip Blumstein and Pepper Schwartz's definitive 1983 study *American Couples*, which showed that lesbian couples have sex less frequently than other couples at all stages of their relationships—during the first two years, years two to ten, and after ten years or more. In the first two years, 33 per cent of lesbian couples were having sex three times a week or more, compared with 45 per cent of heterosexual couples and 67 per cent of gay men.[5]

Gay women in Australia show similar low levels of activity. Dr Juliet Richters from the University of New South Wales recently found that only 37 per cent of lesbian couples have sex once a week or more, compared with 67 per cent of women in heterosexual relationships.[6]

There's much debate as to why this should be. Some argue that societal pressures condition all women to repress and ignore sexual feelings, and the impact of this socialisation is magnified in a relationship involving two female partners. Others believe that bed death is the result of the difficulty women have in being sexually assertive or taking the lead in initiating sexual activities with a partner, a view which is challenged by Suzanne Iasenza, Associate Professor of Counselling at John Jay College of Criminal Justice in New York. In her essay 'The Big Lie: Lesbian Bed Death', she says the evidence shows that gay women don't hang back—they are more sexually assertive, sexually arousable and verbally and non-verbally communicative about sexual needs and desires than women in heterosexual relationships. The result is that they have more orgasms, she boasts.[7]

That's true, says Juliet Richters, whose data showed that 69 per cent of women having sex with a man climaxed the last time they had sex, compared with 76 per cent of women having sex with another women.[8] Women do it better—that is, when they actually feel like genital contact. But as Anne Peplau and her colleagues from the University of California explain in their 2004 review of gay sexuality: 'There appears to be a paradox in lesbian relationships. On the one hand lesbian relationships may increase the likelihood of orgasm. On the other hand, many lesbians emphasize their enjoyment of non-genital kissing and cuddling, activities that are not necessarily associated with orgasm'.[9] Peplau suggests that the greater frequency of sex in heterosexual couples may be due to the male partner's greater level of desire and willingness to take the initiative—which means he ends up pushing the pace. That push is missing in lesbian relationships so the result is lesbian bed death, where genital groping falls by the wayside but cuddles and kisses retain their attraction—a scenario likely to appeal to many women, not only those with gay inclinations.

Well, what about gay men? It is often assumed their double dose of testosterone would result in a sexually charged coupling—and that's just what happens, but only at the start of the relationship. The high level of activity in the first two years— 67 per cent having sex three or more times a week—was very clear in Blumstein and Schwartz's *American Couples* survey. But after a decade of togetherness, only 11 per cent of gay male couples were having sex this frequently, compared with 18 per cent of heterosexual married couples and 1 per cent of lesbians.[10]

Therapists working with gay men report that tensions can arise when the men experience a drop-off in desire after the passing of the limerence stage (that early 'in love' feeling). With male gay culture reinforcing the image of gay men as 'sex hounds' who can't get enough sex, many gay men struggle with self-esteem and identity issues when they find themselves in a less sexual relationship. Many look elsewhere for a new spark—most gay relationships are not monogamous—yet the research finds that the issue of sexual exclusivity doesn't affect relationship satisfaction or the stability of gay relationships. The men are often very sexually experienced when they enter a relationship and are often content in it, even if they find they are not sexually compatible with their partners. As Blumstein and Schwartz explain: 'As their relationships matures, they concentrate on preserving its emotional dimensions. They cease to worry about finding a partner who is the perfect choice sexually. Like the lesbians, they come to feel that the relationship is more important than its sexual limitations'.

Gay men and women march to very different drums and their sex lives reflect the contrasting characteristics of male and female libidos that so often create tension in heterosexual relationships. Lesbian women may well prefer to eat chocolate. But with gay men, the comforts of monogamy tend to be insufficient to curtail that lusty male sexual appetite.

the *Atlantic Monthly*. She describes the Monday night ritual of two of her lesbian friends:

> They order an extra-large cheese pizza (sixteen slices). While waiting—and I am not making this up—they settle in on the couch with large twin bags of Doritos. Each chip is dipped first in Philadelphia cream cheese and then in salsa. Cream cheese, salsa. Cream cheese, salsa. Cream cheese, salsa. The Doritos are finished to the last crumb and then, upon arrival, the pizza as well.[11]

Tsing Loh adds that the couple has an agreement that this night of a million carbs is, by special agreement, guilt-free, and that both feel it is better than sex.

It's fine if both partners come to prefer a good book, or any book, to sex, or see mountains of Doritos as far more desirable than green squares. It's when they don't agree that sex therapists talk about 'desire discrepancy disorders'—it's the gap between desires that's the real problem. Perhaps unsurprisingly, I didn't have any couples happily reporting bed death, lesbian or otherwise, although one couple in their fifties, who had been married for thirty-four years, reported they were both happy with their low sexual frequency. 'Everything else in our relationship is good: we get on extremely well and are still loving partners and enjoy each other's company. Sex is not a huge issue and we tend to laugh the lack of lovemaking off a bit', the husband wrote, mentioning that one might give the other a quick feel in the shower along with the quip, 'Well, that's your lot for the week'.

But Eros loomed large for most of those who volunteered to write diaries for me. Some, like Michael and Heather, wanted to celebrate their good fortune—lusty couples were keen to tell others just how good it can get. But for many, many more, sex had become the elephant in the room, the source of huge amounts of marital tension.

Alan from Townsville wrote to me only once, to tell me his marriage had ended. It was sex that killed it. 'The elephant finally filled the room and left no space for the relationship', he wrote, explaining that he and his wife had suffered years of tension over discrepancies in their desire. They were together for thirteen years, seven of them before marriage. He was left with no idea as to how he could have rescued the relationship after she lost interest in sex:

> I was never one to push the idea of being sexual as I wanted my partner to be in the mood. My partner, however, was never in the mood and was of the opinion that sex was a mutual process where she had to be aroused and interested before it could be initiated. I stopped initiating because I saw little point in asking when I knew she would say no.

So they drifted apart. He writes sadly,

> I found by not being sexually intimate with my wife, the intimacy of the relationship waned. She became a friend and co-parent. We were very infrequent lovers and without being lovers the intimacy part of the relationship was lost. Once the resentments build[s] up the friendship has to be very strong to be able to sustain the relationship. I found my partner very appealing—to have that in front of you and out of reach is frustrating.

He adds that he always loved and respected her. 'I look back and wish I had spoken up more and tried other ways to build the relationship. I paid the price as the relationship ended.'

I have dozens of such letters from people whose relationships ultimately broke apart as the tension grew and grew. 'I thought of it as the "gulf war"', writes another separated man, describing the chasm that grew between him and his partner as they fought over sex:

She felt pressured and I felt frustrated. Mostly she went along with sex, albeit unenthusiastically. I remember one time she said, 'Come on; let's get this show on the road. Forget the foreplay; let's get this thing over with'. Now that is how to make a bloke feel wanted. I didn't know whether to laugh or leave.

Ted, now remarried and happily romping on his Queensland mango farm, tells a similar story: 'I remember in my previous marriage, lying in bed 6 inches from my wife and feeling the gulf between us may as well have been a thousand miles'.

So many of the couples writing diaries for me were caught up in that struggle. Perhaps that's not surprising, with those in trouble being more likely to volunteer, hoping for something to change, than those sailing happily along. What was encouraging was the discovery that some had been there but had found their way through it, bridging that mighty chasm and coming together with their partner again.

Russell (aged fifty-two) is a builder, living in Perth. He's been married to Jess for twenty-six years. His story is fascinating:

> Everything was pretty much running to what we thought was a normal relationship for the first few years of our marriage. The day-to-day highs and lows which come with every partnership trying to build a good family base didn't alter having sex on a regular basis. As years passed, though, things became more and more trying: work loads, bills, normal domestic challenges, not to mention the bottomless wants of our two teenage kids. That played a very big part in our sex drive and by the time they reached their mid teens, sex was a non-event. I can remember not having sex for over a year.
>
> Jess and I reminisce now in bed from time to time over what we were both thinking during those years. She says, 'Some nights I wanted you so badly but didn't know how to approach you'. I had a similar problem towards her. It all stemmed from the fact that we never ever spoke to each other about sex.

Finally, their children left home and found their feet, to the immense relief of the parents:

> This peace of mind has no doubt paved the way for a much rejuvenated sex life. We didn't just decide to get this sex thing back on track; it all happened naturally, and in time. For the past two years Jess and I have never talked so much about sex and now practice and enjoy this lovely art four to five times a week.
>
> A few years ago at the start of our rebuilding process I mentioned to Jess that we shouldn't let our age become an issue with having lots of sex. 'Sex for both of us should be on tap', I told her. We now have an unwritten rule that we never refuse each other's desires.
>
> Initiating sex from both of us is as simple as cuddling in bed. A mere putting your arm around the other is a kind of 'I'm available' gesture. Rejection usually isn't an issue, unless, of course, we are not feeling well or some sort of dispute has occurred during the day. Jess more times than not ends up hitting the sack before me; I usually have extra things to do and she likes to watch TV in bed. Often when I finally retire I find her asleep and don't like the idea of waking her when I'm in the mood. A simple solution—we put one of the small scatter pillows between the sheets as an indication that you want to be woken. Works a treat. I can't help thinking I have a pretty good deal at the mo', in fact very good. That would have never happened five, ten, even twenty years ago.

What was surprising was that the process of writing a sex diary was also a catalyst for this type of change. I quickly discovered that the keeping of a diary seemed to help people to start to think through what was happening to them. Stephanie (aged thirty-four) writes that the day she started keeping her diary, her husband, Anton, saw her doing it when he got home from work and asked what it was about. 'I told him. I counted down from thirty in my head. Sure enough: "So, speaking of sex, any chance of some hot loving tonight?" This is Anton's standard line, and I hate it. It's easier to give in than to have an hour-long argument so I told him yes.'

'Would you like something to put in your sex diary?' became a running gag between many couples, a new saucy type of foreplay. But often the diary writing did more than that. Even when only one person had volunteered for the project, once the other knew they were being observed, it led to changes in their behaviour. They became self-conscious about their actions, a little more considerate, more tuned in to what was happening within the relationship. And couples often started to talk, prompted by encouragement from me.

Look at Nadia and Bill. Nadia wrote to me in despair, complaining that she no longer felt she had a sex drive at all. She'd been married for only four years, and had two young children. Her husband runs a small Sydney transport company; she helps in the business and looks after the children. This 41-year-old woman hated what was happening to them:

> We had a great courtship and had sex a lot like any new lovers. I wanted to be kissed and touched all the time. But after the children came things changed. I felt that at the end of the day, after giving to the children all day, I just wanted to be by myself or sitting with Bill and not touching. After about a year it was very clear my sex drive wasn't coming back any time soon so I went to counselling. It was helpful, but I didn't get any magic answers. My sex drive is zero and I really only do it for him. I know it must be in my head because I was a very sexual person before kids and I can't believe something so drastic changes in your body after kids. I love my husband very much and if there was a pill to take I would take it in an instant.

Her first diary entries are more about avoiding sex than having it.

Tuesday, 3 July 2007—Nadia's diary

Husband is away so I am safe for a couple of nights. Don't think about sex but do use the vibrator because it feels good and I don't have to put out. It's just for me!

Bill was equally miserable, bewildered that their great sex life had changed so much: 'Our courting stage was magical. Fantastic sex, love was mutually expressed very early and we both felt we were the luckiest couple to have each other'. But now, only a few years later, he feels they are floundering: 'I felt every time I tried to hug her I was pushed away. She felt I always was trying for sex. As a result of this I felt rejected, unwanted and unloved. I felt we were going down a path of falling out of love'.

His first diary entries are grumpy and minimal.

Tuesday, 1 August 2007—Bill's diary

Woke up feeling deprived and a little annoyed that on Saturday night Nadia could put across that she is sooo sexy but that is not the case when we are at home. Need to have a pull. Have a magazine in the truck so I pulled over to relieve sexual frustration. Felt a bit desperate. Had to tell Nadia as I handed the soiled jumper to her.

For Nadia, writing a diary means she has sex on the mind. And things start to change.

Sunday, 12 August 2007—Nadia's diary

After a whole night of being poked in the back or stroked in that 'special' way and constantly having to hit him or smack him, I woke up with sex on the brain. I guess because of this diary I must be thinking about it a lot more. During the morning he took the kids out and I decided that when they went down for their sleep I would arrange a little picnic for the both of us and then we could have sex. It was the first time in a long time that I have instigated it at all. I think Bill was surprised and very happy.

A month or so later they are still struggling, but talking a little more honestly.

Monday, 10 September 2007—Nadia's diary

We have been on holiday and I did make more of an effort to have sex. But what our issue is now [is] Bill doesn't just want me to give him sex, he wants me to WANT sex. We had a big fight last night but at the end we both calmed down and talked really honestly about our feelings. He feels that he doesn't feel wanted or loved because I don't [want] to have sex with him any more. He wants it to be like it was before kids but I don't know how to get back to there. But what I did say to him last night was he doesn't seem to try any more. He doesn't shave for days; the romance has all but dried up. He used to be so romantic, always thinking up new ways to say I love you, but when we collapse into bed at night and I get the hand up the leg, he gets NO because I just feel like it's something more to give to someone else. It's like he tries knowing that he is going to get rejected. It all seems to be a catch 22 situation. I don't want to just feel like I am the after-thought at the end of the day.

Then an interesting note from Bill arrived. He'd been out with his mates at the pub. A number of them had young babies and he had listened to them talking about their wives not giving them sex:

Although last time I wrote I said I thought the sex drive was Nadia's problem I now know it isn't. I know it is my problem too. Hearing the way my friends talked really made me realise how closed-minded it is to think it is all your wife's problem. Next week I will try an experiment. I will try to be as romantic as I was when we were courting and see if it affects our sex life and how it affects our relationship.

Next came a worried little letter from Nadia—Bill had read some of her diaries! 'I didn't mean for him to read my letters to you. I feel terrible. I re-read the one he had and it would have been so hurtful for him to see that. I guess I must have been angry when I wrote it. Anyway I hope I can make up for it this weekend.'

Yes, he was hurt and this wasn't part of the plan. The couples were supposed to keep their diaries private. But in this case, it seemed to help achieve a breakthrough.

Wednesday, 24 October 2007—Nadia's diary

Things have definitely turned and I think it is a combination of what we have talked about and also what Bill read last week. He has not pestered me for sex at all. The wandering hand has not had to be kicked away. But instead we are mutually responding to 'something'. When we are sitting last thing at night I give him a foot massage. More cuddles are going around. He bought me flowers, I bought him flowers!! More text messages during the day of love and things like that. We have had sex twice and once instigated by me and once sort of instigated by him, but not forced on me. It was one morning, quite early. In my head I was saying I should instigate sex. But it was only 5.30 a.m. ... and I was still unconvinced that I actually wanted to wake at this time. But when his hand was on my leg I just moved so it went elsewhere and one thing led to another. We were disturbed by our four year old—thank god for DVDs and Thomas the Tank Engine!—but it ended up being very nice. I didn't feel forced and he didn't feel like he had to beg.

Many of the women writing diaries were finding that if they could get their head into the right place and instigate sex, it really helped them to enjoy it. It gave them a sense of agency which helped to restore their sexual confidence, as Nadia was finding. Bill and Nadia are not out of the woods yet, but their future is looking a lot more hopeful.

Monday, 29 October 2007—Nadia's diary

A great week I think has been had by both of us. I did my first real initiation of sex and it went something like this!! Bill was leaving very late for work on Friday, which is very unusual—he's usually gone by 6 a.m., but he didn't have to leave till 8.45 a.m. He was getting dressed and I had just jumped out of the shower. One child was in the bedroom playing and the other one was watching a DVD, so I grabbed Bill and asked if he wanted a quickie. He laughed and we were rolling around on the bed. He wasn't getting hard and I asked what was going on. He said he had a lot on his mind—work, the kids, more work. I said, 'You're not going to say no, are you?' He replied, 'No, of course not, but I don't know if it's going to work'. We both laughed because it was as if the shoe was on the other foot. Anyway, it worked and he left for work a happy man and me a contented wife, so pleased that I was able to do that.

Saturday was a very nice day. The kids went off to their sleepover in the afternoon and we went out on a rented kayak —something we used to do before kids. We then came home and I went off to the gym while Bill had a sleep. We went out for dinner and came home to have very drunk[en] sex!!

Again more sex in the morning, not so drunk. We were taking advantage of no little feet coming into the bedroom. It was very nice. I must say that even though I am sure Bill instigated the Saturday night and Sunday morning there was no resentment, no angry feelings. He has been very careful not to grope me or to just fondle me at the end of the day. I think something is working and I like it.

There has been a complete shift in the way Bill and I are communicating. Firstly he has stopped groping and pawing at me for sex. And because of this he has opened the door to allow me to make the first move. He is still in shock and walks around with a smile on his face. He feels that I want him again, our desire for each other is growing. It was something so small but it has made a huge impact on our relationship.

A year after they first started writing for me, Nadia reported they were now far happier:

> I wouldn't say we are having more sex than a year ago, but I definitely am trying to instigate or at least not slap him away every time he wants me and I feel that Bill doesn't seem to be groping as much and pestering me all the time. Of course there are times when this does happen but we can point it out to one another and talk about it. We have got so much better at talking about the way we are feeling and what is going on for both of us. If we find we are slipping back into the old ways we can talk about it and try to do things to fix it.

But she's still disappointed that spontaneous desire is now a thing of the past:

> I must say that I am sad to read that my sex drive may never come back to the way it was at the beginning of our relationship. It seems to be a cruel thing that 'mother nature' or whoever has played on us women!! I am still hoping someone will come up with a little pill and save the day for women so we can keep up with the men and feel great at the same time.

For women who have known what it is like to really want sex, losing that drive is a mighty blow. Again and again, women told me that they wanted it back. As Nadia explains, 'I guess it comes down to I am still waiting and wanting my sex drive to come back and I want to enjoy sex again. I know that we are much happier but I still want to have the WANTING feeling'.

3

Where Has She Gone, This Lover I Married?

> He can't cuddle me without 'accidentally' touching my arse or
> my breasts. It always feels like a grope to me and a 'how about
> it' feel. Most of the time he just gets smacked away but every
> now and again I feel bad for him, so sad that he is rejected all
> the time.

The grope. It features regularly in so many of the female diaries.
Women complain about cringing when their partners cuddle and
then hands wander uninvited across their bodies, touch their
breasts, feel and fondle. The grab at the breasts as they pass in
the kitchen; the grope under the skirt on the way up the stairs.
Listen to this woman: 'This morning I was in the shower when he
left for work; he came to kiss me goodbye, which was lovely. But
he had to rub me on the vagina, which drives me mad!'

I started to talk to the men about this, asking them if they ever
groped, and what it was all about for them. Sydney man Clive is
forty-eight and has been married for twenty-two years in a stable,
happy relationship. 'We still love each other very much. The only
real issue is sex', he says, explaining that his wife is only interested
in sex every week or two, whereas he would love it twice a day.
'On the face of it, it appears we have the perfect marriage. Maybe
I hide my unhappiness too well.'

Clive is a self-confessed groper:

Oh, yes. I admit to it. A caress of the bottom, the arm, her hair, her breast (caress rather than squeeze), her back. Sometimes I'll caress the outside of her pubic bone. Sometimes at night over recent years I've even taking to sliding my hand into her panties while she is asleep and just touching her pubic hair. My fingers can just feel it and she knows that is as far as it will go if she stirs a bit. We both know it won't lead to anything.

I try hard to not exceed allowable limits. To sense her mood. I wonder whether us men are sometimes the more sensitive sex. We seem to have a lot of practice at it. Grope too much and you'll be 'off sex'. So you must do it carefully. It's almost like being a young man and trying to work out how far your girlfriend will let you go before the shutters come down, she crosses her legs and says NO.

I know that a caress won't get me any sex. So it's more like, 'I love you, I'm desperate for you. Just touching you is a connection from me to you. I'm still here. I still adore you. Hullo! Where has she gone, this lover I married?'

Where has she gone, this lover I married? This cry from the heart captures men's deep yearning and sadness that the magic they once shared with their lovers has disappeared, and the despair that they feel at the prospect of spending the rest of their lives grovelling for sexual favours.

That was perhaps the most fascinating aspect of the sex diaries—to hear these male voices talking about what it was like for them. So many of the men told me that this was the first time they had ever talked openly about what was happening to them in their sexual relationships, about how it affected them. They have all tried to talk to their partners and have often met a rough reception. 'Sex, that's all you ever think about', the women say scathingly.

Clive gets quite indignant at what he sees as unfair treatment. 'For years we men have been lectured about PMS. How we should understand about women and their hormones and moods. Maybe it's time women started to be lectured and understand about ours', he writes, explaining that when he becomes really frustrated and irritable, sometimes his wife will notice and ask what's wrong. 'I tell her I've got LLS (lack of love syndrome)!' he says, adding that 'sometimes that gets a sympathetic laugh or giggle which helps somewhat'.

That's the thing. The women complain that men never stop thinking about IT, and the men are left feeling there is something shameful about wanting to make love to a lifetime partner, about yearning to caress the woman they have married. It is not just about sex, the men respond.

They are right. In his book *What Could He Be Thinking?*, Michael Gurian explains that levels of the bonding chemical oxytocin are normally far lower in males than in females, but that this changes at orgasm, leading men to associate sex with a strong emotional connection:

> When a man ejaculates, he bonds utterly with her. One of the primary reasons that men want sex more than women (on average) is because it feels so good to them to have the high oxytocin—it feels great to feel so bonded with someone. All humans get an explosion of joy, fun brain chemistry—oxytocin being a major player—when we achieve bonding. In male biochemistry, sex is the quickest way for a man to bond with a woman.[1]

So one major reason why men want sex more than women is that it feels great to have a high oxytocin level, to feel so connected to someone else. Women can have that feeling all the time; men need to have sex to achieve that intense emotional bonding. Cut off from sex with a loved partner, men yearn for that ultimate connection.

'I just feel so lonely', writes Patrick. The 43-year-old Townsville man sends a photo showing his arms around his pretty wife, Sue.

They are both smiling—his head inclines towards her, big brown eyes twinkling. 'We get on really well, we don't fight or argue, but when it comes to intimacy, or sex, she doesn't want to know. I love her dearly but it seems more like we are brother and sister or friends.'

Arthur (aged sixty-three) is a Perth doctor who has been married to 'B' for over thirty-seven years. His diaries make such sad reading, filled with stories of love and unrequited lust: 'I would just be another dirty old man if I were having these thoughts about a woman to whom I was not committed. But she's my wife of many decades. I think I'm just an old romantic'.

Thursday, 1 March 2007—Arthur's diary

To bed together, unusual for us: my wife has refused any sex at night for more than fifteen years. She says she can't sleep after sex. I sleep very well of course.

She: 'I am aching all over. Everything hurts.'

Me: I reach out to stroke and soothe her but she has wrapped the blankets around her so tightly. I can't touch her.

She: 'What do you want?'

Me: 'I want to touch you, to stroke you.'

She: 'Just leave me alone, let me sleep.'

I feel disappointed, rejected, sad.

Friday, 2 March 2007

I wake up before her. We have to get up soon and go to work. I reach out—she leaps out of bed and says, 'I have to go to the toilet'.

Me: 'When you are finished come back and make mad, passionate love to me.'

She: 'Ha, ha!'

Two minutes later she does come back, dressing gown over nightie. I persuade her to cuddle into me. It's pretty awkward and not at all sexual.

Monday, 5 March 2007

I am seated in our bedroom, putting on my shoes. As usual, time is short. She comes out of the shower and stands before me, naked. She says, 'Are you ready to go?' I say, 'Yes, unless you want to come over here so I can give you a head job'. Her reply is just 'Har har har!' I long for her body but she has avoided oral sex for a year or two. The rest of Thursday is just a flat-out rush until late at night.

This is not just about men wanting to get their rocks off. Craig (aged forty-five) from Cairns writes that 'the wonderful rush of love and closeness that you get when making love is like stepping stones through the turbulence of the other aspects of your life together'. For most men it is about making love. But for many it is also about wanting to be wanted; wanting to be desired by the woman they love; wanting to feel like a real man, a man who is a successful lover.

Look at Mac, forty-four years old and from Broken Hill. He's been married for twenty-one years to Lesley: 'A great lady and a fantastic mother'. She is forty-two and still a very attractive and desirable woman, he says.

To start with, sex was wonderful: 'We were like rabbits, two and three times a day, especially on weekends. She was often the instigator'. Then came the dip:

> The last five years has seen the dip take a dramatic effect. From about four to five times a week to maybe once every six months. She started off by using the 'You are getting more than the average guy' [line] to now just offering excuses of too busy, too tired. We don't discuss it at all now. Get it over with as quickly as possible. She hasn't kissed me passionately for five or six years. When she touches me it feels to me like she thinks I am dirty, no loving touches any more, again leading to my feelings of failure.

He's overwhelmed with the feeling that he has let her down. He deals with it

> like anyone deals with an addiction. I loved sex a great deal with my wife and have been and will continue to be faithful. I feel I have failed her needs in the bedroom and that has soured her interest. Now I go out of the way to avoid temptation near me. I do not shower with her, or see her naked.

Faced with her lack of interest, his reaction is to tiptoe around her, deny his needs and avoid confrontation. How different is that from the past when sex was simply part of women's 'wifely duties', when a man was free to claim his conjugal rights? Clearly such patriarchal marital arrangements led to some atrocious behaviour. But now the pendulum has swung far in the opposite direction, perhaps too far. Most men find themselves on the back foot, feeling very much at the mercy of women's whims. And that means the whole business of seeking sex has become very hard work for men.

I once saw a very funny performance by San Francisco comedian Tom Caylor about why men like pornography. There's a man lying in bed. Beside him is his wife—gorgeous, available, warm, loving, naked. But what's he doing? He's reading a sexy novel, getting his kicks from the little black dots marching across the page. Why, you ask? Oh, he knows exactly why:

> Because, see, if I wanted to have sex with her, I would have to put down my book, I would have to roll over, I would have to ask her to put down her book, I would have to say, 'How are you doing? Are the kids in bed, is the cat out, is the phone machine on, are the doors locked, maybe we should brush our teeth, is the birth control device handy?' Then I would have to turn on the sensitivity, I would have to ask her what's been goin' on with her, what she's been dealin' with, I mean with the kids and the house and the budget and her mom and everything like that.

> I'd have to tell her what was happenin' with me. My problems, my worries. I would have to hold her, I'd have to stroke her, I would have to commit myself to an act which these days I may or may not be able to consummate. You think that is easy? The little black dots, they are easy.

The skit brought the house down. People recognise the shift that has occurred in relations between the sexes. They get the message that the power to reject is now firmly in the hands of women. But is this just because so many women end up being less interested in sex? David Schnarch, in his influential book *Passionate Marriage*, makes the point that the spouse with the least desire for sex always controls it. They are the one who sets the rhythm and pace of the sexual relationship. The other partner may nag and cajole, but the power lies with the one saying 'No'.[2]

It's certainly true. With couples where the woman has a much stronger drive, it is the man who controls the pace of lovemaking and the women don't like it at all. Miranda (aged twenty-five) from Sydney had been living with her partner Harry (twenty-seven) for only a few months when she first started writing for me, but already they were running into problems over sex:

> I'm still fairly regular in my libido and Harry has commented previously that I don't seem to ever subside even when I'm working fifty-two hours a week and attempting full-time study. I seem to have a stronger drive, [but] when he's been working late or is sick his drive just seems to die in the ass and I get frustrated with him.

It was obvious early on that she was struggling with always having to be the one to make the approach:

> I was thinking about how rejected I feel when I come home from work and molest him only to get a groan and him rolling away from me. I feel rejected by him a lot of the time; we are quite different. Sometimes he just doesn't feel like entertaining

my advances, pushes away my embrace, retreats from my touch and makes a whingey noise when I'm trying to make a connection. It annoys and upsets me.

And then suddenly came the note from Miranda to say they had split up. This young woman was one of ten female diarists with notably stronger drives than their partners. Four of the ten left their partners over the six to nine months during which the study was conducted.

The numbers are too small for any real conclusion, but it was striking that these women took action when confronted with an unfulfilling sex life while so many of the male diarists were simply putting up and shutting up. It speaks of an even more important change that has taken place in male–female relations—a dramatic reversal of power. Over the past few years, there's been a seismic shift in relationships away from the patriarchal authority of the past. And men know the ground has moved beneath them.

Some fifteen years ago, social researcher Hugh Mackay was already reporting changes in the state of play in Australian marriages, noting the Australian male's 'dim awareness that something has gone wrong with his life'. This dim awareness was summed up by one of Mackay's male interviewees as follows: 'Years ago, a lot of women were scared to go crook at their husbands, but now the men know that if it is bad enough and they don't take notice, the women could leave'.[3]

With their new-found economic independence topped up by the promise of welfare support, women gained the power to leave unhappy relationships, and that changed everything. Previously, women were forced to make the most of their marriages—dependent on their husbands to provide for them and their children, they had no other choice but to stay put. But now the rose-coloured glasses have been tossed aside and women judge their relationships much more harshly. They expect more and are in a position to act on their convictions.

This has led to women's discontent with their relationships becoming the major factor in our divorce rate. In countries across the Western world, women are the ones who make the decision to leave in two-thirds of all marriages.[4] 'Slam! That's the sound that one million US men hear each year as their wives push them out the doors of their homes and into the divorce courts', begins Brown University psychiatry professor Scott Haltzman's recent book *The Secrets of Happily Married Men*, making the point that the US divorce rate has escalated from 14 per cent to nearly half of all marriages, with women initiating most of the separations.[5]

The heart of the problem is the often unrealistic expectations women have for their relationships—their desire for intimacy, for greater emotional reciprocity in their marriages—and, particularly for women with strong drives, the assumption of a satisfactory sexual life. 'In the end, we are left with an extraordinarily heightened set of expectations about the possibilities in human relationship that lives side by side with disillusion that, for many, borders on despair', writes US sociologist Lillian Rubin.[6] In the early 1980s, Rubin was one of the first to document women's dissatisfaction with the lack of emotional connection in their marriages. She found that women yearned for their men to supply intimacy based on the shared feelings and confidences that traditionally enrich women's relationships with each other.

'It is undeniable that women, on the whole, are less satisfied with marriage than men are', says La Trobe University sociologist Ken Dempsey, whose work on emotional satisfaction in marriages evolved out of research on housework. He found that many men and the great majority of women see marriage as offering a better deal to men—with housework and childcare issues central to the perceived inequity—and that women are far more vocal in listing the causes of dissatisfaction.[7]

John M Gottman is one of America's foremost researchers on marriage. In 1999, he published an intriguing study which tracked

130 newlyweds, carefully observing how the couples interacted with each other and then following up the research for six years to see which marriages were happy and stable, and which ended in divorce.

Gottman and his colleagues recorded their surprise at the outcome:

> Men should forget all that psychobabble about active listen-ing and validation. If you want your marriage to last for a long time … just do what your wife says. Go ahead, give in to her … The marriages that did work all had one thing in common—the husband was willing to give in to the wife. We found that only those newlywed men who are accepting of influence from their wives are ending up in happy, stable marriages.[8]

The researchers suggested that this was a fairly recent develop-ment in marriage dynamics, coinciding with 'the loss of power [in marriage] that men have experienced in the last 40 years'.

So now it is men who are more emotionally dependent on their relationships—they are the ones choosing to bite their tongues and put up with unsatisfactory sexual relationships in order to stay with the women they love, and to avoid losing their families. It seems that Skyhooks were right when they sung 'All My Friends Are Getting Married'—men really are doing what they're told.

Doing what they are told means tiptoeing around the missus in the hope of keeping her happy. Diarist Clive talks about trying really hard to help around the house to make sure his wife doesn't get 'too tired' and avoid getting into arguments, because if she got angry then there would not be any sex for the next week or more: 'When you're on survival rations, every little bit counts'. Another man once talked to me about trying to decide if it was worth having a fight with his partner over a television program: 'We always watch what she wants to watch. So what I have to decide is, is it worth having an argument over the telly, risk getting her in a bad mood and giving up any hope of getting any sex?' But doing what they are told may also mean going for years, many years, without sex.

Wayne is a 66-year-old Darwin man, married for forty-five years and with what he calls a reasonably high libido. He reports that, apart from the first year or so of marriage, his wife has always been trying to make excuses as to why she couldn't have sex: 'About twenty years ago she found a way of avoiding it altogether, by either going to bed before I did, so that she was sound asleep when I went to bed, or she waited up until I went to bed and was asleep before she would come into the bedroom'.

Finally, he decided to take a stand. About eight years ago, he made a statement that he now acknowledges to have often regretted—'I'll make no advances or ask for sex until you ask me'. And the result? 'In the last eight years there has been no sex in our marriage at all.'

Lest you think this is unusual, I received many similar stories when I talked publicly about Wayne's situation. The sex drought in Craig's home, for instance, has lasted five years:

> The last time we had sex she obviously did not enjoy it, and she got up the instant I had finished to go and wash any trace of me off her. Her manner and extreme reaction made me feel like I was dirty and worthless, the kind of reaction I imagine a hooker feels towards her clients, and this deeply affected me. I vowed I would not be the one to institute sex again, that it had to come from her, when she really wanted it. It's been nearly five years since then and still no approach from her.

I have heard from so many men who are just hanging in there, year after year, wishing and hoping. Yes, some men do leave, but what is striking is how many more stay, knowing what they are missing but determined to stay put. They often write so movingly about their regret over how their relationship has fallen so short of what they had imagined. Anthony, a 47-year-old Bathurst man married for eleven years to 51-year-old Adele, writes:

> It seems like we are living in black and white in a high colour world, all for want of removing the monochrome glasses. I can accept this if I have to, but I remember colour, and I know what a joy it can be—I want to share that with her.

Anthony says he has discovered that he can live with a low sex drive, 'but it is far from my first choice'. The couple has had long periods without sex—'gaps of years, and many, many months'. And when they do have sex, it is very different from what he really wants:

> Adele is not someone who enjoys any stimulatory sensory contact—she loves a cuddle, being close, static touching—but not a caress, a tickle, erotic massage, or any form of what to me would be passionate holding in lovemaking. When we do make love, we do not have foreplay, she is embarrassed or put off by any form of romance, but she is quickly physiologically ready for sex, and usually achieves orgasm. To me it is businesslike and mechanical—it is OK to laugh at this point, because we seem to be the reverse of the stereotypical couple!

And yet this is a strong marriage and he never thinks of leaving:

> We have a fantastic relationship—we are both thoughtful to each other, we have never yelled at one another, or had an argument (although we have had difficult discussions of course); no one has ever needed to 'sleep in another room' or storm out. There is plenty of love between us—emotionally if not physically.

Sex or no sex, most men are willing to stay because they love their wives and children and they know how much they stand to lose if they leave. And some aren't convinced they would end up any better off if they did change partners. As one young man wrote after a failed relationship: 'As for the future, well I can't ever see myself getting married if I have to resign myself to a life of begging for sex. It's far worse being in a relationship and not getting any than being alone and getting the occasional shag'.

In Kate Grenville's novel *The Idea of Perfection*, bank manager Hugh Porcelline gets a surprise when his wife, Felicity, poses naked for amateur photographer and local butcher Alfred Chang. Hugh is determined to carry on as if nothing has happened. His only comment on the incident concerns their son's awareness of his mother's adventures—'Just not in front of William, darling'. The two don't talk about what has happened. 'They had never talked about it the other times, either. There was no point. You just put it behind you.'[9]

Note the modern twist in the story. Now it is the man, rather than the woman, who is turning a blind eye to a partner's unacceptable behaviour. In previous generations, women were the ones who were forced to put up with whatever cards were dealt to them in a marriage. Now it is men who are clinging to their relationships, choosing not to know.

What is striking about Grenville's portrayal of Felicity is that she is well aware of her power to exploit her husband's dependence: 'Just for that moment—the space of a breath—she knew how unbearable it was for him … She saw how it was her—the choices she herself was making—that was inflicting it on him. Just for one puncturing moment she saw herself: a cruel smiling child'.

I once spoke to a man whose wife had contacted me when I asked for volunteers to discuss marriages that have survived affairs. Pam told me that she'd discovered Leon had had an affair while she was pregnant with their first child. After a stormy period, her husband's affair died out and Pam took up with her next-door neighbour Dennis out of vengeance. 'I thought, "Damn them, if they are going to do it, I'll do it too".' So she did, and the affair was in its nineteenth year by the time I spoke to her.

Pam was sure Leon knew the affair was still going on. But when I finally talked to him, it quickly became apparent that he was not working on that assumption. Leon told me, 'I was devastated when the affair started. She was quite open about it. I'd be going off to squash and she'd say, "Oh, Dennis is coming around tonight". But it's over now. Oh, I know she's no longer having an affair. I think it only lasted a few months'.

Listening to this man talking about what he called 'the best years of his life'—the past decade when his children were growing up—it's clear he's very glad he decided not to run off with his lover. He wanted his marriage to last. And now he has the good sense not to rock the boat by asking sticky questions.

Men, now, are sticking it out, making the best of their situations, turning a blind eye and, when they have to, putting up with sexless marriages—living in relationships that fall well short of their dreams.

Of course, often I am hearing only one side of the story. Many of the more miserable male diarists had partners who absolutely refused to take part in the research. 'Sex research? Oh, for goodness sake. Why don't you grow up and act your age', one woman told her husband. Yet it could be that these women also feel they are missing out. Perhaps some of these men are expecting the world and giving little—failing to pull their weight at home or show the consideration and sensitivity to her needs that would prompt the sexual generosity they so sorely desire. But there's also no doubt that women now feel entitled to close up shop. Safe in the knowledge that they are no longer under any obligation to put out when they are not in the mood, sexual rejection easily becomes a way of life.

For the rejected men, the grope is still there, a symbol of all their lost hopes, a reminder of what they once had. 'What is now considered a grope was once just a special hug that only you two could give each other—and I don't mean going for gold in the knickers. Maybe just an arm around her chest, something only I was allowed to do and not sexual at all', explains Craig. He knows the grope is now out of bounds, but sometimes he forgets: 'I get a rather violent flick of my arm away from her. Shame. It's those moments of close cuddles, embrace, that I miss as much as the sex. In fact I would probably be able to cope a lot better if they were still there instead of the brush-off'.

Another diarist, Sam, sums it up: 'Men remember when their wives couldn't keep their hands off them. I got married thinking marriage would create more opportunities for affection, romance, sex and exploration. It's nice to feel wanted, desirable. When wives start to refuse their husband's advances men become confused and emotionally hurt'.

Women switch rules in the middle of the game and that simply doesn't seem fair. 'Why is the same bloke who was once a desirable red-blooded male now considered a groper, an inconsiderate molester? What changed? Who changed?' Sam asks.

It is women who have changed. The old saying about marriage has never been so apt: 'Women hope that men will change after marriage but they don't; men hope women won't change but they do'.

4

The Search for the Elusive Pink Viagra

It's easy to find women who have a low sex drive. They are everywhere. A recent television news item in Adelaide announced drug trials involving women with low libido. The researchers were stunned by the response to their call for volunteers: 1500 women from all over Australia. 'It was incredible', said Professor Robert Norman, one of the researchers.

Lack of sexual desire is the number one sexual problem plaguing women today. Over half (55 per cent) of all women experience lack of desire according to the *Sex in Australia* survey, a research project involving nearly twenty thousand participants, which makes it one of the largest sex studies ever completed.[1] The researchers, Juliet Richters and her colleagues, found that low libido isn't simply a problem that affects older women—over half the surveyed women under thirty had the same complaint. Women in their thirties were most at risk, with over 60 per cent being uninterested, which was fractionally more than the oldest category of women surveyed (aged fifty to fifty-nine). Women in their forties did a little better at 55 per cent.

So we're talking about a problem that can affect women from the very start of their adult lives, women like Sophie from Wollongong. She's a student, aged twenty and married only eight months when she first contacted me—eight months and she'd already gone off sex. 'I'm not sure whether my decline in libido is a result of too much of a good thing, or whether I'm just instinctually bored with the same old partner', she writes. Her 'same old partner' is aged twenty-two.

Here's one of her first diary entries:

> My libido over the past few days has been at zero. I don't know whether it's the Pill, or stress, or if I'm just un-horny. Poor Dave is just about pulling his hair out. I worry that he thinks it's because I don't love him as much or find him as attractive any more. This isn't the case. I'm just finding sex a bit passé. Even a bit annoying at times. The most unfair part is that his libido doesn't seem to have declined at all! He swears blind that every time feels like the first time, and literally has never said no to sex.

This is a woman who is only twenty, just married. While I did hear from lusty women who have retained their sexual drive throughout their lives, their numbers were thin compared with the women reporting low libido. Women of all ages complained they were not interested in sex. Some said their libido dipped soon after they settled in to a relationship, while others found that their interest held up but then nosedived when they had children. Another group of low-drive women said they were never very interested. What's going on here?

In my view, the reason so many women have such low sexual drive is simply to do with the way we are made. Women struggling with this problem often mourn their lost libido. 'Why did I go off sex?' they ask themselves, remembering the times when they were always randy, wanting it, longing for it. That was the Real Me, they tell themselves. But perhaps the horny woman was the aberration that masked their true nature. Now they are stuck with the normal female libido—fragile, delicate, distractible and rarely lighting their fire.

The truth is that sex experts and researchers really don't know what is happening here. Many believe that women's low drive is linked to their low level of testosterone; women have ten to twenty times less of this vital hormone than men. Testosterone is responsible for male characteristics such as facial and body hair, deeper voices, more muscular bodies. We also know that testosterone is strongly connected to libido in males—testosterone-deficient men lose interest in sex. While we think of testosterone as the definitive male hormone, it is also produced in women by the ovaries and synthesised in other regions of the body—body fat and skin, for example—from the hormones DHEA and DHEAS. So women have testosterone too, but in smaller doses. The meagre supply may be one reason why women's libido is such damp wood, lacking that chemical spark that keeps so many men interested in sex.

But as the eloquent Natalie Angier makes clear in her book *Woman: An Intimate Geography*, our knowledge of neurobiology is still primitive. We don't understand how hormones work on the brain to elicit desire or feed a fantasy or muffle an impulse. Angier argues that humans are intelligent, thinking, emoting animals and, as such, hormones are unlikely to ever be more than a tiny part of the picture.

> The greater the intelligence, the greater the demand on the emotions, the portmanteaus of information, to expand their capacity and multiply their zippers and compartments ... Hormones are part of the suitcase and part of the contents. They relay information about themselves and they carry information about others. They do not make us do anything, but they may make the doing of something easier and more pleasurable when all else conspires in favour of it.[2]

In light of this, it doesn't seem to make sense to try to reduce any individual's sexual behaviour to a particular hormonal condition.

Social relationships, cultural and family values and future aspirations have a far stronger influence on sexual behaviour than sex hormones alone.

What makes matters even more confusing is that many women remember times when they were consumed by lust. 'I couldn't keep my hands off him. In the first three months, sex was constant, nearly every night, sometimes two or three times a night, if I wasn't too sore', says another twenty year old who wrote complaining that after six months in her relationship, she was totally indifferent to her partner.

The explanation for this early interest may be that the damp wood is given a mighty dose of firelighters through the rush of brain chemicals that are released when we first fall in love. These are the so-called infatuation chemicals—epinephrine, norepinephrine, dopamine, serotonin and phenylethylamine (PEA)—neurotransmitters which help regulate the electrical signals between nerve cells in the brain. It's these chemicals that cause the emotional high associated with that glorious madness of first love—what the French call *le coupe de foudre* (the lightning bolt).

Lightning bolt is right. I'll never forget the dinner I shared with my first husband, Dennis, the night we fell in love—gazing at each other transfixed, unable to eat. The waiter hovered, asking whether there was something wrong with the meal. There was glorious anticipation, heart-stopping intensity and total lust.

Dopamine is the main cause of the sexual sizzle, suggests Rutgers University anthropologist Helen Fisher, who has scanned the brains of wildly infatuated people, tracking the dopamine activity associated with those delicious feelings so familiar to many of us. Fisher and her colleagues took snapshots of brains in the throes of infatuation using functional magnetic resonance imaging (MRI) technology. Lovesick students were scanned while they looked at a picture of an acquaintance and again while gazing at a picture of their sweetheart. When researchers compared the images, they found increases in neural activity in the parts of the brain rich in dopamine. Students who scored highly on a questionnaire measuring passionate love showed particularly increased activity in the caudate nucleus, a passion-related region of the brain. 'The giddiness, that elation, that euphoria, that sleeplessness, that loss of appetite, is associated with high levels of dopamine, and norepinephrine. These are natural stimulants in the brain that give you feelings of elation', Fisher explains.[3]

But here, too, chemistry is clearly only part of the story. When two lovers first come together, there's the incalculable thrill of the new—all that yearning, longing and then, finally, the moment when lips meet, hands touch for the first time, a new body, exotic scents and sensations, all wrapped up in the rosy haze of romance. How can we tease out the psychological impact of the novelty and excitement of these experiences from whatever chemical buzz we might be experiencing at that time?

Whatever the mix, the result is that heady, early 'in love' feeling—what psychologists call limerence—which often has a powerful effect on a woman who ordinarily has little interest in sex. She'll find herself fantasising about sex, initiating sex, behaving like a person with a high sex drive. Many of my female diarists remember these heady days of their relationships as a time when they thought of themselves as driven by sex. They wrote to me saying that they used to love it, want it all the time, when they were crazy with love.

It was marvellous reading the diaries of the couples still steeped in limerence—like Kevin and Amanda from Melbourne. They were my newlyweds. Well, actually, they weren't even married when they first started writing for me, but by the end of the process they were engaged. Both were in their early thirties and had been married before, and they had been together less than a year when they started writing the diaries. Yet they were the couple who best captured the newlywed spirit, consumed by lust for each other, madly in love and delighted to tell me all about it.

It's a typical night in September 2007. Kevin arrives home from work; Amanda is preparing the dinner. He runs a bath for her five year old and, with the boy happily splashing with his bath toys, returns to the kitchen to find Amanda bent over the sink, her pants on the floor. 'Let's go', she says to him.

'I just had a thought of him taking me there and then', Amanda writes, explaining that a quick shag at the kitchen sink had become one of their special rituals. Kevin needed no encouraging. 'That's one of the best things about our relationship, the spontaneity. The passion when we just go for it is amazing', he writes with his usual enthusiasm. It was a quickie, as the little boy needed to be rescued from his bath: 'Just enough to whet our appetite for later on'. As the evening progressed, they had trouble keeping their hands off each other, hugging and touching whenever they came close. Kevin explains:

> Eventually we make it to bed, hot with the expectation of what is about to happen. I can actually feel my heart rate go up as I get into bed, in anticipation of Amanda's touch. We make love a second time and it is just incredible. I feel so high when I make love to her: it must be like being on drugs. I feel like I am in a place when I am untouchable, invincible almost.

For month after month, that desire kept going strong. 'Have I mentioned just how much I am in love with this woman? I can never get enough of her, whether it be hugs, kisses, just touching hands, or the amazing love that we make', writes Kevin.

Amanda is less effusive on paper, but clearly very happy to participate in their active sex life. Here she is, in her own quiet way, describing a typical encounter:

> We got into bed, spent some time kissing and touching. I was very aroused quickly and it was Kevin tonight who said to me

that he was going to take his time. We were very close tonight. Like an invisible energy field wrapped around the two of us. I love it when it is like that. Very intense and all the senses are heightened. I came a couple of times before Kevin and then we lay in bed for a while holding one another.

It is not just the sex. They are very sweet to each other, going out of their way to find ways of pleasing one another. 'It doesn't matter how bad a day I have at work, I always look forward to coming home to Amanda … I am always greeted with a smile, and usually a big hug and kiss', says Kevin. He, in turn, is constantly on the lookout for ways of helping ease her load: doing household chores, cooking dinner, making her coffee. It was such a pleasure to read about this couple's daily lives and share the intensity of their pleasure together.

Eventually, real life did start to intrude. They were trying to conceive and, after a while, her diaries were filled with references to plotting temperatures and the monthly disappointment of her menstrual cycle arriving. They both have difficult former spouses to deal with—he has the added strain of missing his children, who live in another state, and the highs and lows of visits to them. Yet beneath it all was this wonderful, driving lust.

This chemically driven infatuation tends to wear off after nine months to two years. There is a change in brain chemicals, with those involved in attachment—namely oxytocins and vasopressin—becoming more dominant, suppressing lust and romantic love. On the plus side, partners in the attachment stage of love trigger the production of endorphins in each other, providing a sense of safety, stability and tranquillity. But, as Helen Fisher points out in *The Anatomy of Love*, this comes at the expense of mutual sexual desire. This means couples have to work at remaining exciting to one another because 'in some ways you are bucking a biological tide', she maintains.[4]

This drop-off in a woman's sexual drive comes as a shock to the high-drive men who were convinced they had met the woman of their dreams—the woman who could never get enough sex. Sam from Brisbane tells me about being out late one night with friends when he and his wife were courting:

> I decided to be considerate because Anne had to work the next day. Instead of finding somewhere quiet to make the beast with two backs, as would have been normal, I drove her homewards. As we approached her home, she realised what I was doing and asked me why. I told her. 'Silly boy', she laughed, punching my shoulder, 'never too tired for nookie'.

But soon after, Anne, at age nineteen, tried to avoid sex on her wedding night because she was so exhausted after all the endless preparations and the big day itself. 'A smart man would have walked out then, before consummating the marriage, but I was young, dumb and in love. I wonder if I was an unwitting victim of entrapment', ponders Sam. Getting married was like throwing a sexual switch, he reports—the girl who was never too tired for nookie became totally uninterested.

It's not surprising that many men conclude they were deliberately duped. Yet the truth seems to be that Cupid spins his web of limerence, artificially inflating the woman's libido and thus hoodwinking not only the man but the woman herself into thinking she has a strong drive. I am reminded of the heady days in the 1960s when it suddenly became fashionable to live together before marriage. The idea was to have a trial run, to see if you were really suited to each other. 'It's important to see if you are sexually compatible' was the popular line. Now, all these years later, we are discovering how we were conned—trial runs tell you nothing about whether mutual lust will survive.

But we're not just talking about *levels* of desire—women's libido seems to work differently from that of men. Dr Rosie

King is one of Australia's most experienced sex therapists and the author of *Good Loving, Great Sex*, a very good self-help book on problems of desire, in which she sums up the observed differences between the male and female sex drives. The male drive is more urgent, less distractible and more goal-directed, which means it takes a lot more to turn men off sex than it does to turn women off. With women, sexual drive is more diffuse and distractible, and it's linked to emotional connection—all features that social anthropologists conclude are biologically based protective mechanisms which help mothers to care for their young. 'Women are hot-wired so they will never be so overcome by lust and passion that they neglect their major responsibility—the well-being of their offspring', says King.[5]

But there are other differences. In her book *Women, Sex and Pornography*, Melbourne writer Beatrice Faust contrasts the *sexual styles* of men and women, reaching the depressing conclusion that 'much of the time men and women do not seem to be complementary or even compatible'. She discusses research showing that females are more sensitive to touch, with baby girls having a lower pain threshold than baby boys, and more rapidly develop greater sensitivity; female babies are also more sensitive to the removal of coverings and exposure to a jet of air. Male babies are less tactile but grow up to be more readily aroused by visual stimuli—they respond more to erotica or pornography, and by observing the opposite sex. Male sexuality is more easily conditioned—it is rare for a woman to acquire a sexual fetish where her interest is directed towards objects rather than her partner. Men are somewhat aroused by the trappings of sex—sexy underwear, suspenders, long boots, high heels—and it is predominantly males who develop the uncommon sexual practices which usually show a history of sexual conditioning.[6]

The result is that men go to bed with their imaginations. Their sexual appetites are stimulated and sustained by a whole range of erotic images and events which have gone before or may happen in the future. In his book *Sexual Behavior in the Human Male*, Alfred Kinsey talks about the differences between male and female sexual drives, which result from the male's ability to be conditioned by his sexual environment. The male goes through life picking up and responding to all sorts of visual erotic clues which feed his sexual imagination. He then parcels these up and takes them to bed with him—an instant source of arousal which exists totally independently of the rest of his world, including his relationships.[7]

This makes men very versatile. They may prefer intimacy but they don't need it in the same way that women do. They can settle for raw sex, with no side dishes. Remember that old joke about men not needing to look at the mantelpiece while stoking the fire? Well, many men are able to respond in trying circumstances, to women they find unsympathetic or unattractive. They can use their imagination to light their fire and keep them sexually on heat.

'I cannot remember a time when I was so stressed, tired or anxious that I did not want sex. In fact, if I am emotionally stressed, tired or anxious, sex is without doubt the best relaxant', writes 48-year-old Clive. He adds that he knows exactly why a certain former US president got into trouble: 'From a male point of view, I can understand why Bill Clinton got a blow job in the oval office. With the weight of the world on his shoulders, the best relaxant had to be a sexual orgasm'.

If there's strain in Clive's relationship, he's convinced that sex is the best way to relieve it: 'If things aren't going well, I want to make love to her, as it is my most intimate moment'. But for his wife, it is different. For her, the argument has to be dealt with first—'an emotional rebuilding period before sex re-emerges, which comes with the reconnection of the relationship', Clive explains.

Both men and women wrote to me, fretting over these differences. 'If he has just yelled at the kids, I stand there and wonder how I could ever have sex with him again', writes Phoebe (aged thirty-six), explaining how anger at her husband turns her off sex:

> Larry wouldn't care if I had just been horrible or if we weren't getting along; sex would always cheer him up. His answer to everything is sex—it would cure a cold, a headache, a bad day, fix an argument and yes, I think it is an escape for him.

But this Melbourne couple have learnt to live with the differences between them. 'When it comes down to brass tacks, my husband and I have come to the annoying conclusion that we are wired differently and we have agreed to try not to take it personally', she says, reporting that sex is lower on her to-do list than 'sleep, exercise, running the house, looking after the kids and keeping the mental and emotional train that is our family on track'. She remembers reading a women's magazine article when she was in her mid twenties which talked about women thinking of the laundry while having sex: 'I remember being puzzled and thinking, "As if!!"' A few years later, she was doing the same.

Even when she was at her hottest, Phoebe always wanted sex 'to be part of a whole. Unless I was drunk or feeling particularly reckless, I wanted sex to be at the end of a dance that included mental and emotional twists and turns, and I would prefer to have a long, non-sexual massage first'. She adds that she always responds better if she is relaxed.

Recently, Larry was using some macadamia nut oil during cooking and asked if she would like him to rub it all over her. 'You're kidding. On a Sunday afternoon with kids in the next room?' was her immediate reaction. She told him that if he were to take her to a special weekend retreat, then she'd like it:

> I felt it was a bit sad, that to do something that could be relaxing and fun, I needed to be transported, wined and dined

and I did feel a bit mean and dry and crusty. But the truth is I would prefer to be away from all the distractions of my life so I could fully enjoy sensual, slow and relaxing sex rather than have to fit it into an already crowded mind and over-demanded body.

That's what I hear from woman after woman—that their men don't understand why they need everything to be just right to want sex. It's not that they are particularly unhappy with their partners. It's just a simple fact of life that most of us live in imperfect relationships, in which we confront daily irritations and stresses which pile up and swamp that fragile female libido. Just think about it—Phoebe's husband yells at the kids and she finds herself wondering how she will ever have sex with him again. Doesn't that say it all?

It is hardly surprising that research trying to pin down factors affecting libido in women always cites relationship problems as one of the major passion killers. But what's crazy is the assumption in the sex research literature that all women with low drive have troubled relationships.[8] Surely it makes more sense to conclude that it is normal for the female libido to be a casualty of everyday relationship stresses than to assume that this huge number of women—more than 55 per cent—is stuck in deficient relationships? Yes, some of my diarists are clearly miserable and others are very aware that issues from their past, including sexual abuse, continue to cripple their desire and sexual response. But many other female diarists report that their low desire creates a rare thorn in an otherwise pretty harmonious partnership.

What emerges very clearly is the conflict between men and women over their differing needs for intimacy. Most women need to feel close to their partners to want sex. When I talk to women about what this means, they often say they require some concrete gesture, some connection to his thoughts and feelings. 'I want to know what he's thinking, what's going on inside him, before we jump into bed', they tell me.

For women, intimacy tends to require talk. In *Intimate Strangers*, Lillian Rubin writes:

> For the woman, intimacy without words is small comfort most of the time. It's not that she needs always to talk, but it's important to her to know what's going on inside him if she's to feel close. And it's important to her to believe he cares what's going on inside her.[9]

Rubin describes how difficult that demand for verbal intimacy can be for men. She found it was a common experience to ask a man 'How does that feel?' and see a blank look on his face. Yet this type of intimate talk, this exchange of feelings, is second nature for many women.

With women, the demand for intimacy seems bound up with high levels of the bonding chemical oxytocin, the brain chemical that controls maternal nurturance, verbal-emotive connection and empathic bonding. Women have higher levels of this chemical than men. Hence, while testosterone pushes a man to desire physical contact, oxytocin makes emotional connection the priority for woman. As I mentioned in Chapter 3, the only time male oxytocin levels approach the normal female level is during orgasm. Michael Gurian explains this in his book *What Could He Be Thinking?*: 'Testosterone and vasopressin, which got him to the point where he could successfully achieve coitus, receded in dominance—their job complete—and oxytocin, the bonding chemical, took over'.[10]

So these basic differences in brain chemistry seem to underlie that gulf between men and women in their approach to sex and intimacy—that men want sex in order to feel close to their women, but women need to feel close to their men in order to want sex.

Having said all that, we shouldn't forget that sometimes it is the man who is less interested in sex or who needs an emotional connection in order to want sex. While all these male/female differences involve commonly observed patterns, there are exceptions to every one of them. As we will see in Chapter 6, there are men whose sexual response also follows the twists and turns of an emotional relationship, and men who have very low libido. There are also women who retain their sexual drive and even those for whom it gets stronger.

'Now I know how good it can be, I want it more', says Trish (aged forty) from Adelaide. She reports that she didn't enjoy sex much as a young adult: 'In my twenties I was with a lot of men who didn't know what they were doing. They needed to be taught and I didn't know what to teach them'. She's very frustrated now to be with a great lover, her husband, who's not very interested in sex. 'Now I know what I have been missing and want to make up for all those wasted years in my twenties! I would have sex every day if I had a chance.'

We know so little about why these patterns occur and why there are exceptions to the rules. What research exists often simply confuses matters. Even the basic question of how many women have low drive proves difficult, with some sexual surveys estimating only 7 per cent of women are in this situation, while other surveys put the figure nearer to 60 per cent. It all depends on how they ask the questions. In the *Sex in Australia* survey, researcher Juliet Richters and her colleagues asked how often women had experienced loss of desire for *at least one month in the previous year*. Fifty-five per cent of the women responded positively.[11] A group of Melbourne researchers led by Richard Hayes came up with a similar number (58 per cent) when they asked that exact question, but almost half that number (32 per cent) when they asked about low drive *in the previous month*.[12]

Such differences in defining low drive explain discrepancies in the international results, the researchers explain.

Hayes and his colleagues went on to look at how many women were actually upset by the problem, a combination of low desire and distress that had been labelled 'Hypoactive Sexual Desire Disorder' (HSDD). When they looked for women with HSDD, the figure dropped even further, down to 16 per cent. It's fascinating that many women experience low desire but that this only bothers some of them. US women, for example, are more likely to be upset by low libido than women in Europe, and, as women get older, they are also less likely to be concerned about low drive.[13]

A huge controversy has blown up in recent years, with sex researchers and therapists battling over whether it makes sense to talk about a desire 'disorder' if so many women aren't concerned about their low drive. Leave them alone, say the critics, concerned that the current worldwide interest in women's low libido is being fuelled by drug companies keen to follow up on the dramatic success of drug treatments for impotence with a pill for libido. Australian journalist Ray Moynihan is among the most rabid critics. He has made a career out of arguing that pharmaceutical companies are doing the work of the devil. In 2005, in *The British Medical Journal*, he took aim at efforts being made by sexologists to differentiate and carefully define female sexual problems such as lost libido, lack of orgasm and pain in sex under the new label 'female sexual dysfunction'. Moynihan claimed the sex researchers were conspiring with drug companies in the 'corporate-sponsored creation of disease' to create new markets for their products.[14]

Others have similar qualms. Leonore Tiefer, a clinical associate professor at New York University School of Medicine, also argues that these female sexual problems are being oversold with the backing of the drug companies. 'Ever since Viagra proved to the pharmaceutical industry that contemporary sexual confusions and dissatisfactions could be medicalized and marketed (to the sweet cash register ring of billions of dollars and Euros), companies have been searching for some way to make women into sex problem consumer patients', she writes.[15]

One result of this criticism has been a push to regard low libido as a problem only if it bugs the woman herself, which brings the numbers right down. However, most of the women writing to me about this issue are concerned not because it bothers them to have little drive, but because they worry about the impact on their relationship. And that's fair enough. Think about the problem of the man who can't control ejaculation. When we have a guy who is trigger-happy, we'll talk about 'premature ejaculation' because even if it doesn't bother him to come really quickly, it may mean his partner will miss out on pleasure. The impact on the relationship is a big deal, making what therapists call 'desire discrepancy' a very real issue.

So it absolutely makes sense to keep searching for a magic bullet for women, although there won't be a pink Viagra. While Viagra and similar drug products which increase penile blood flow have revolutionised the prospects for impotent men, it is now clear that increasing activity in the loins isn't going to make any difference to sexual desire for most women. In 2004, the pharmaceutical giant Pfizer gave up research into women's use of Viagra after discovering that even though these drugs resulted in greater genital blood flow, many women didn't even notice. Pumping women's genitals full of blood simply didn't make them frisky. 'There's a disconnect in many women between genital changes and mental changes', commented Dr Mitra Boolel, the leader of the Pfizer research team.[16]

But the search continues. There were plenty of women among my diarists who would pop a pill if they knew it would work. Many had already wasted money on herbal remedies that promised to lift libido—to no avail. That's what's so infuriating. Everywhere there are snake oil salesmen who are making a fortune by ripping off women who are desperate for a boost to their libido.

Or snake oil saleswomen—like Sonia Amososa. She's the young, blonde Australian company director who was named a few years ago on a 'Young Rich List', with her company valued at a cool $38 million and growing fast.[17] Her 'libido enhancer'—Horny Goat Weed—is one of the company's best sellers. The product is a mix of herbs with fancy names like *Epimedium grandiflorum, Smilax officinalis* and *Theobroma cacao*, plus assorted vitamins—products for which there have been no safety tests, no clinical trials, no guarantees you aren't buying a lemon. Horny Goat Weed has repeatedly been reported to the Therapeutic Goods Advertising Codes Council, which found no evidence that the product did enhance libido. But the only result was that the company now has to take care with their advertising. Your sexual function *may* be improved, says the sneaky fine print in the more recent ads.

Rest assured, if any of these herbal 'libido-boosters' contains ingredients which actually work, the pharmaceutical companies are onto them. One 'nutritional supplement' which recently received a proper trial is ArginMax, which contains L-arginine, ginseng, ginkgo, damiana, multivitamins and minerals. About half of the women involved in the drug's research trials showed a boost in sexual desire when taking it. One of the researchers is a major player in the sex research field, Beverley Whipple, a former president of the American Association of Sex Educators, Counselors and Therapists, who suggests that, while more research is needed, this product shows some promise.[18]

Of all the current possible magic bullets, the best candidate is testosterone, which seems to work effectively for some women. Yet as a hormone, it will never have the direct, rapid effect that Viagra has on men. Female testosterone levels gradually decrease with age—women in their forties have blood testosterone levels which are, on average, half those of women in their twenties. In particular, low levels of DHEAS can be associated with low drive—women with low sexual function are three to four times more likely to have a DHEAS level in the lowest 10 per cent for their age, according to researchers at Monash University.[19] Yet there are also women with low levels of this hormone who have a strong libido. The situation is complex and, as yet, there is no good diagnostic test to decide who would benefit from treatment with testosterone. A trial run using testosterone is often the best way to determine whether it will make a difference.

'It doesn't help all women. Approximately one in two women show benefit but for some it makes a substantial, really meaningful change', says Susan Davis, Monash University's professor of women's health and a world leader in hormone research. Davis has overseen projects in eighty research study centres in Europe, the United States and Australia, supported by the drug company Proctor and Gamble, and has demonstrated that testosterone boosts libido in post-menopausal women (including those who are menopausal due to the surgical removal of their ovaries) and, more recently, also in younger, pre-menopausal women.[20]

Some experts feel it is premature to use testosterone in therapy to address low drive, particularly given concerns about the long-term safety of the drug. Although many medical practitioners routinely measure testosterone levels to determine who should be given the drug, the latest research suggests that this type of testing is not helpful. No one really knows what level is appropriate for treatment. 'If you are treating a 50 year old, do you bring her up to the normal range for a woman of her age or treat her to bring her up to the normal range for a younger woman? No one has sorted this out', comments Davis.[21]

Sydney sex therapist Dr Margaret Redelman, who has been assisting in the trials of testosterone, agrees that the issues are confusing. 'I have seen women with very low testosterone levels with good libidos and women with high levels who have poor libido', she says, stressing that hormone levels are only one of a complex range of factors contributing to low desire. But she has been using testosterone as part of a range of treatments for ten to fifteen years and finds that for some women it makes a real difference. 'It doesn't make you want to jump anybody. But women often have more sexual thoughts, feel more willing to engage in sex, and have more energy, a sense of well-being', she says, adding that this can be a big deal for women distressed about their low libido.[22]

I spoke to Yvonne (aged fifty-two), a Melbourne academic whose depression led her to seek out Professor Susan Davis— she'd read a newspaper article reporting that Davis had found that depression in menopausal women is sometimes caused by low testosterone levels. Sure enough, Davis found that Yvonne's levels were very low and put her on the testosterone cream, Andro-Feme.

'I felt like I used to feel when I was twenty. My energy levels were up. My sex drive went *boing*. The testosterone fired me up', Yvonne told me. The change was amazing. Within a week she noticed not only a shift in her mood, but that her dampened sex drive was now up and running: 'I had always enjoyed having a really high libido. Now it was back!' And six years later she is still reaping the benefits. Davis is carefully monitoring her progress but Yvonne is determined to stay on the treatment. 'I don't want to give it up. I feel fantastic', she says.

There have recently been successful trials of an as-yet-unreleased testosterone spray. Women using the spray experienced much more pleasurable sex and very few side effects.[23] (Too much testosterone can lead to masculinisation, including excess body or facial hair, oily skin, acne, scalp hair loss and enlargement of the clitoris.) The spray treatment is soon to be the subject of a large-scale trial in the United States, to properly evaluate its effectiveness and the safety issues. Work is also underway on testosterone skin patches, gels and lozenges.

Professor Davis sees it as critical that all the testosterone treatments receive such rigorous evaluation. A few years ago, the US Food and Drug Administration decided that more study was needed before Intrinsa, a testosterone patch for women, could be released on the market. That's fair enough, says Davis, but she points out that Viagra was released onto the US market without any of the long-term safety information now being asked of the female products, and with a very similar level of effectiveness— an interesting double standard. Testosterone implants have been approved for use in the UK, but the only form of testosterone treatment approved in Australia for use by women is Andro-Feme, and it can be used only in Western Australia, where it was developed. Off-label methods being used to treat women include testosterone pellets, which are surgically implanted in abdominal fat, as well as tablets, lozenges and injections developed for men.

For women who are keen to find something to boost their libido, testosterone is well worth a try. Meanwhile, the search for sexual wonder drugs for women goes on. More precisely targeted drugs are on the drawing board which don't light up the entire nervous system in the blind hope of hitting pleasure buttons, but home in on the parts of the brain that are directly connected with arousal and orgasm.[24]

There's a group of scientists studying the specific areas of the brain involved in female orgasm, working on the assumption that female sexual response has more to do with what happens between the ears than between the legs. One of these scientists is Dr Gemma O'Brien, a physiologist from the University of New England.[25] Her research on the neurobiology of orgasm focuses on the role of oxytocin—'the cuddle hormone'—which she feels might be a key player in desire and arousal. O'Brien believes that there may be a genetic reason why certain women enjoy sex less than others: 'Many genes regulate all the different things that happen during sex. Maybe some women have less active genes for producing oxytocin, or for driving desire'. Since oxytocin is important for connecting with partners, she suggests that if we could switch on the oxytocin genes, a woman's interest in having sex with her partner might return. There is evidence from twin studies, both from Britain and Australia, that up to half of the variation between women in their ability to climax is due to genetic factors.[26]

O'Brien proposes that 'differences between the genes that produce steroid hormones in women would explain some of the differences in women's responsiveness when treated with oestrogen or testosterone and the ways that hormone levels alter at menopause'. The key sex hormones—oestrogen, progesterone and testosterone—belong to the class of chemicals called steroids. Some tissues of the body have enzymes that can transform one steroid into another. 'Genetic differences would influence the activity levels of these enzymes in different women,' suggests O'Brien, 'leading to differences in libido and sexual enjoyment'.[27]

Another piece in the libido puzzle is menopause, which effectively wipes out sexual drive for many older women. The Melbourne Women's Midlife Health Project has found that as women pass through menopause, there's a significant increase in reported sexual problems, such as low sexual drive and responsiveness, vaginal dryness and painful intercourse. According to Professor Lorraine Dennerstein, who runs the project, the major culprit is the drop in levels of oestradiol (the main form of oestrogen). 'As [oestradiol] falls, down goes your desire, down goes your arousal, down goes your response', says Dennerstein.

Hormone replacement therapy, or HRT, helps some women regain their drive, but with testosterone levels often having fallen in this age group, sometimes testosterone proves more effective.[28]

Susan Davis has recently completed research on a menopausal drug called Livial. It contains tibolone, a synthetic steroid that has been found to increase women's natural testosterone, resulting in increased sexual drive, energy and sense of wellbeing.[29] Since Livial also offers the benefits of other HRTs, such as reducing hot flushes and preventing vaginal dryness, the drug may be a good option for post-menopausal women who notice a drop-off in sexual drive.

There's something else that can bring back the sexual zip for women after menopause—a love affair. Dennerstein's research finds that sexual desire, enjoyment and arousal all snap back into action when women find themselves with a new lover. This shows that hormones are only a tiny part of the story, says Dennerstein. 'Far more important is what's happening in your relationship. If you find a new feller at this time or feel more loving towards your partner, that will overwhelm the effects of oestrogen loss.'[30]

But for how long?

Rachel, a 55-year-old Canberra bureaucrat, steamed through early menopause fuelled by lust for her new lover, Roger:

> I seemed in a constant state of lubrication. He is a wonderful lover. I would just have to think about him or receive a phone call or email or text message and I'd be ready to jump into bed with him. We wouldn't wait to have sex at any time anywhere.

Roger (aged forty-six), a medical researcher, was at the end of a 20-year marriage which had been sexless for the last seven years. He writes with such joy about meeting Rachel, 'the partner I had been looking for', and their three wonderful years together. He says their relationship is incredibly supportive and loving, with high levels of libido and intimacy. This is a passionate man clearly rapt in making love to his adored partner:

> I'm quite addicted to giving Rachel orgasms. I love it that I can please her, that she says I'm good at it and that it makes her feel good to be touched that way. I love touching her—the physical sensation—and because she takes a little while to climax, it just means I get to touch her for longer. And—this may sound crazy—I love her smell and taste which sometimes stay with me for hours.

However, by the time Rachel first started writing to me, she had gone off the boil. She never felt like having sex any more. 'I feel like I'm enduring sex most of the time', she said, adding that she normally still reached orgasm due to Roger's loving efforts:

> Roger would probably still like to have sex twice a day but twice a month sounds good to me. When we've had sex I'm relieved because it'll be at least a day before the pressure is on again. I haven't been honest with Roger about this because I know he will be hurt and that's the last thing I want. I love this man and want to spend the rest of my life with him. I am distressed about the sex situation and I wish I could enjoy it more for his sake. He tries really hard to make me feel beautiful and sexy.

As they write their diaries, they gradually talk more. Roger acknowledges that he was devastated when Rachel confessed to him that she was no longer interested. It is very sad seeing in his diaries how the worry over Rachel's low interest starts to eat away at his pleasure.

Tuesday, 20 November 2007—Roger's diary

Yesterday I had quite a day puzzling over recent events between Rachel and I. Over breakfast I got the distinct impression that

I'd done something wrong by giving her an orgasm [the night before]. My mind wandered to recent conversations about our differing libido and Rachel getting too much sex. So by the time I walked home I was in a bit of a mood. We talked a little, quite an emotional discussion. At one stage Rachel said that if she were asked how often she would like sex she would say never. It was difficult to take and despite discussing it we were both moody all night and slept badly.

I've also been thinking about Rachel masturbating me and the 'wifely duty' thing. It's lovely of her to do it—I don't know what percentage of the partnered population would be so thoughtful. But I don't want her to feel compelled—to do it out of duty. The selfish side of me wants her to want and enjoy doing it, but perhaps those days have gone.

Rachel is a joy to be with. I love her personality, her character. I'm watching her now planting some flowers in the front yard and doing some weeding. I'd rather masturbate every day than be without her.

As they talk more, they become tense with each other. Rachel suggests that maybe the solution includes having 'quickies', telling him it would be fine by her to have intercourse sometimes without feeling the pressure of having to respond. But he says that for him, that would be like asking a racehorse to give pony rides to children. At this time intercourse was off the agenda because she was recovering from one of her frequent urinary tract infections (UTI), which often follow intercourse.

Wednesday, 21 November 2007—Roger's diary

It's a quandary for us both now. At home it feels like we're treading on eggshells. It's a little tense and emotional and I'm reluctant to bring anything up for fear of spilling over the emotions and upsetting Rachel. And just what do we talk about anyway? Rachel has no libido—wants sex never. I have a relatively high libido, want to be intimate with her, and want to experience with her all the things I feel I've missed out on in life. In bed this morning we hugged a little and I gave her a rub on the back, careful to make it caring and not doing anything that might constitute a sexual advance.

Friday, 23 November 2007—Rachel's diary

I feel as though we are living in a sexless household now. The relief I felt for a moment is overshadowed by a deep sadness that our relationship is forever changed. I feel awful for Roger. He is being so kind to me and I know he is terribly hurt. There is a glimmer of hope, however. I went to the Sexual Health Clinic this morning and my hormone levels are being checked. I may go on the contraceptive pill to pick up my oestrogen levels. Hopefully the flushes will reduce so I can get some sleep and my libido will pick up. He's not looking at me and is not touching me as much, although he put his arm around me this morning in bed while I was naked. That made me happy.

They have had the good times, their glorious period when limerence wove its magic and turned Rachel into the lusty wench of Roger's dreams. Now they face reality and their diaries reflect all the tension and heartbreak that comes when two people who love each other no longer share the same mutual desire.

But five months later things start to get better, the tension begins to ease. Rachel's HRT means she has fewer infections, and the hot flushes have disappeared so she's sleeping better— and more likely to be in the mood for sex. She says, 'I have had a psychological shift in my attitude to sex. Now that I'm not so terrified of UTIs and because Roger is so sweet and considerate in not pressuring me into having sex too often, I can really look forward to the inevitable, wonderful orgasm he will give me'.

Roger says he is over his intense disappointment at discovering that Rachel's libido was floundering. 'I'm hoping she is not feeling pressured into having sex. I'm getting less sex than I would like but I can live with it knowing I am with the woman I love', he says, adding that he has his fingers crossed that they might one day return to the sex life they once had.

Some time later I received another note from Roger, with a postscript. They had just had their wedding anniversary, which included dinner in an elegant restaurant followed by an overnight stay in a chic hotel. Rachel turned up to the dinner dressed in her wedding dress. 'She looked so beautiful', Roger writes. After dinner they returned to their room, which Roger had lit with candles.

> What surprised me was Rachel's attitude to sex that night. She was quite the aggressor—throwing off inhibitions and concerns. Under her dress she wore the pearl thong I had given her a year or so ago and she let me know about it! We had sex like we did in the olden days. It was lovely.

So Rachel is having fun throwing off her inhibitions and initiating sex, at least on special occasions. But she freely admits another big change—she now realises that she doesn't need to want sex to end up enjoying it. 'I know that even though the desire is not there to begin with, it won't [take] long for my body to respond to his touch and I can enjoy the delicious feeling of arousal and feeling close to my gorgeous husband', she writes.

This couple has come a long way. It was so worrying to read their diaries when Roger discovered Rachel's loss of desire and struggled to deal with that knowledge. The tension between them was palpable. It came as a relief when they seemed to turn the corner, partly as a result of Rachel's discovery that she could 'just do it', comfortable in the knowledge that in the right hands, her body would respond. That has turned out to be one of the real keys to sexual harmony—not only for Rachel and Roger but for couples everywhere.

The chances are that a magic bullet for women will one day appear. The pharmaceutical companies are bound to come up with solutions when so many women are crying out for drugs to boost libido. But even more important is the need for a change in women's thinking, accepting that 'just do it' is part of the answer.

5

Just Do It!

On 20 July 1969, Neil Armstrong, the commander of Apollo 11, became the first person to set foot on the moon. His first words—'That's one small step for man, one giant leap for mankind'—became part of history, televised to earth and heard by millions. But just before he re-entered the lunar module, he added an enigmatic comment: 'Good luck, Mr Gorsky'.

Many people at NASA thought it was a casual remark concerning some rival Soviet cosmonaut, but a check revealed there was no Gorsky in either the Russian or US space programs. Over the years, many people questioned Armstrong about what he meant, but he always just smiled. Then, on 5 July 1995 in Tampa, Florida, a reporter again raised the question and this time Armstrong responded; it seemed that Mr Gorsky had died and so Armstrong felt he could finally answer. He explained that, in 1938, when he was a kid in a small Midwest town, he was playing baseball with a friend in his backyard. The ball was hit over the fence and landed in the yard of the neighbours, the Gorskys, by their bedroom windows. As Armstrong bent down to pick up the ball, he heard Mrs Gorsky shouting at Mr Gorsky. 'Sex! You want sex?! You'll get sex when the kid next door walks on the moon!'

It's a great story but, sadly, only an urban legend—one which regularly does the rounds on the internet. But how fascinating that the Gorsky story so perfectly captures the start of a new era. Neil Armstrong stepped onto the moon just at the time when women's sexual rights were becoming a rallying cry. Women must no longer act as spittoons for men, preached Germaine Greer, calling for an end to women's sexual subjugation. After all those years of thinking of England, now women could reclaim their bodies for their own pleasure, and that meant having sex only when they felt like it.

Female desire must come first, pronounced New York sex therapist Helen Kaplan, as she adapted sex researchers Masters and Johnson's famous 1966 model of sexual pleasure to make desire the prerequisite for all that followed.[1] Without desire there was no arousal, no pleasure, the experts pronounced, and feminists applauded.

As terrible stories of marital rape and sexual violence began to claim the public's attention, women's right to refuse sex became fundamental to decent relations between the genders. It became a total no-no to ever suggest that women should be pressured into sex. Remember Justice Bollen? In a 1992 marital rape case, this South Australian judge blundered into dangerous territory when he suggested that 'there is nothing wrong with a husband, faced with his wife's initial refusal to engage in intercourse, in attempting, in an acceptable way, to persuade her to change her mind, and that may involve a measure of rougher than usual handling'.[2]

Rougher than usual handling? Of course, the sky fell in over these unfortunate words but one suspects that even without them, Bollen would have come in for a caning for daring to suggest that men should ever try to persuade women to come across.

The belief was that sex must wait until women are well and truly in the mood. But that was where we went wrong. The assumption that women need to want sex to enjoy it has proven a really damaging sexual idea, one that has wrought havoc in relationships for the past forty years. The sex diaries show that so very clearly, revealing that many women firmly believe that unless they feel like having sex, they can't possibly make love. And the men know that all too well. Many work hard to try to kindle the flame of desire in their partners, knowing that without this they will run into a brick wall of rejection. But it rarely works and couples' sexual frequency falls hostage to women's weak libido. The result is that sex becomes a battleground as sad, rejected men rightly complain when physical intimacy and the consequent emotional connection fall by the wayside.

Amy spent the first ten years of her marriage fighting about sex. 'Every night he'd have a go. He'd reach across the bed and it was my decision whether it was on or not. It was this big ogre between us', says this 54-year-old woman, who lives with her husband, Jim (aged fifty-six), in Hobart, Tasmania. Amy continues: 'Even if I refused him I'd be so upset that I'd lie awake at night thinking, "Why did I say no?" I might as well have let him have it because the next day he'd be so grumpy'. 'That's right', Jim acknowledges ruefully, 'I was a great sulker'. Even on the days he didn't approach her, Amy says she was always nervous. 'He'd be snoring loudly and I'd still lie there worrying that the hand was going to come creeping over.'

It's now almost twenty years since Amy lay rigid in bed, dreading the creeping hand seeking her body. 'I look back and am amazed now that we let sex become such a source of tension between us. It was because we couldn't talk about it', she says. But that wasn't the only reason that the chasm between them kept growing. There was another dilemma—in Amy's head. She was convinced she shouldn't have sex without desire.

As Amy discovered, if she waited for her own sexual libido to rear its weedy little head, the frequency with which the couple had sex became low indeed. After one particularly nasty fight, Jim announced he was sick of having to approach her for sex. 'If you ever want sex again, you are going to have to ask me for it', he told her. 'That was a complete and utter disaster', says Amy, describing how she'd lie awake worrying about not wanting sex, yet knowing how grumpy he'd be if another day went by without it.

Amy finally realised it was the idea in her head that was the real problem—that if she could get over that stumbling block of thinking she had to want it first, she'd enjoy sex and all would be fine. 'It doesn't matter to me whether I'm desperate for sex or not, whether I want it or not. As soon as it gets started it's OK. I'll enjoy it. But that took me a long time to learn', she says. Amy now counsels other women through her church and says that many are extremely resistant to that message:

> They often haven't had sex for years because they say they have no desire, yet they are looking for love and intimacy and closeness to come back. I explain to them that's never going to happen unless they start having sex again. But when I tell them to do it they are often horrified, saying that's like being a prostitute.

But many women find that their sex lives improve immensely if they can get their head around this radical rethink.

Research by Professor Rosemary Basson from British Columbia has shown that many women do experience arousal and orgasm if they have sex without any prior desire.[3] Basson has found that women in long-term relationships may rarely think of sex or experience a spontaneous hunger for sexual activity. So when they do have sex, they are seeking emotional closeness or intimacy with their partners or responding to his overtures, rather than being prompted by their own desire. But even though they may not be 'in the mood' to start off with, once they start making love, these women often feel sexual sensations building, desire may start to click in and then they'll want to continue. The result is that they experience sexual pleasure and perhaps orgasm. Provided there's a 'willingness to be receptive', the rest follows, Basson advises.[4]

'Just do it!' suggests sex therapist Michele Weiner Davis in her bestselling book *The Sex-starved Marriage*. She says that desire is a decision—you can't just wait for it to come, you have to make it happen. She's reached that conclusion as a result of years spent counselling couples who are experiencing tension in their marriages as a result of one spouse—usually the wife—not being interested in sex. What she found was that many reluctant lovers reported that when they did have sex, they ended up feeling good—once they were into it, they were into it. Weiner Davis poses the revolutionary idea that there's no point worrying about the reasons why women aren't interested in sex—there'll always be plenty of them: squalling infants, stress, tiredness, irritation that he won't help with the housework. 'Knowing why you are not so interested in sex won't boost your desire one bit. Doing something about it will', she says.[5]

It seems that many women are willing to do it. They manage the sex supply by sometimes having sex when they don't feel like it. An internet survey conducted by the *Australian Women's Weekly* found that 73 per cent of the respondents reported they do sometimes have sex when they're not in the mood. And half of these women give as their reason: 'I know I am likely to end up enjoying it', followed by a third who do it to keep their partners happy.[6]

Yet the idea of having sex without desire is now considered reactionary, a challenge to the feminist orthodoxy that has ruled our sexual lives for decades. 'To contemporary women, the notion that sex might have any function other than personal fulfillment is a violation of the very tenets of the sexual revolution that so deeply shaped their attitudes on such matters', comments Caitlin Flanagan in her thoughtful *Atlantic Monthly* essay 'The Wifely Duty'. She found herself reflecting on those repressed and much-pitied 1950s wives—'their sexless college years! their boorish husbands who couldn't locate the clitoris with a flashlight and a copy of *Gray's Anatomy!*' Flanagan wonders whether these put-upon housewives might, in fact, be getting a lot more action than many of today's liberated and sexually experienced married women.[7]

It's an interesting thought. We have long assumed that these liberated times have led to a flowering of sexual activity—that couples today are shagging more often and more successfully than their predecessors. But perhaps, as Flanagan suggests, past generations of women considered that sex was part of their wifely duties and so they went with the flow. It's quite possible that many more got off in the process.

As Flanagan explains it, wifely duty meant that 'a housewife understood that, in addition to ironing her husband's shirts and cooking the Sunday roast, she was, with some regularity, going to have relations with the man of the house'. But she questions whether this sex was, as some feminists suggest, inevitably 'grimly efficient interludes during which the poor humped upon wife stared at the ceiling and silently composed the grocery list'. Maybe not. For if the 'just do it' theorists like Rosemary Basson and Michele Weiner Davis are right, some of that sex might not have been all that bad. More likely, suggests Flanagan, when you get the canoe in the water, everyone starts happily paddling.[8]

These days, the very suggestion is enough to give feminists apoplexy. 'Fuck you Bettina Arndt!' was the charming beginning to a blog responding to my writing about the 'just do it idea'.[9] The blog writer, 'blue milk', felt I was suggesting that we shouldn't worry about why women aren't interested in sex any more, but 'just pressure them into it by threatening the future happiness of their families and pretty soon their libido will be bouncing right back'. She had some stern advice for men. 'Do Not Bully Or Guilt Or Coerce Someone Into Having Sex With You! No one owes you a fuck: married, partnered, or single, there's no guarantee in life that your sex quota will be filled', she tells them, suggesting masturbation is the solution for those times when he wants sex and she doesn't.

This chat site quickly filled with the comments of equally angry women. 'It sickens me that after so many YEARS of feminism we are still arguing [for] the most basic of rights—the right for a woman to make decisions about her own body', one hissed.

But 'blue milk' has it wrong. The 'just do it' idea isn't about encouraging women to be subservient to men, nor does it suggest that women suffer through unpleasant, painful sex. I never proposed that if women have more sex, their sex drives will leap back into action. I simply made the point that women who have diminished libidos often still want to have sex for reasons other than their own desire—they want to have sex to feel close to their partners, to make them feel good, AND ALSO because they know it will make themselves feel good too. Many know that if they can get their head in the right place before they start making love, they will enjoy, they will respond, they will get excited and reach orgasm. Once the canoe is in the water, they do paddle happily.

Why is this such an outrageous idea? How is this an inappropriate suggestion in this feminist age? OK, 'just do it' ends up making sex work better for men, but provided it also gives women pleasure, it is hard to understand why it creates such an uproar. If you actually talk to women about this, many will tell you that they do it for their own pleasure, not just to please their partners.

Listen to my diarists. Edwina (aged sixty) from the Gold Coast knows exactly why she just does it:

Firstly, I'm married to a wonderful man and he's very easy to please. So, I decided that even if I couldn't really be 'bothered' to have sex, it would make him happy, so that's how 'just-do-it' began. He did so much for me, so it was the least I could do for him. Secondly, it's good and the initial reluctance always disappears. He's happy and so am I. Simple really. He's never ever pestered me either; I'd hate a man who was 'at' me all the time. That's another reason for me to be 'reasonable' towards him.

'I do love the closeness too', she says, but adds, 'my libido is very low really and if I'm widowed, it won't worry me to totally stop having sex'.

Then there's Glenda (aged forty) from Melbourne: 'I'm definitely a "just do it" person. There may be an odd occasion when I actually feel like it, but I never have any problems once we start. It always feels good and I always wonder why I don't "just do it" more often'.

One particularly fascinating letter came from Claudia, a young woman who explained she was in an arranged marriage. She described spending the early years of her marriage fighting with her husband about sex, but then she realised she might as well enjoy it: 'You have enough chores and responsibilities, why add sex to the equation? Why not make it part of the enjoyment of life, the happiness, the thing you look forward to?' What she now does is 'reprogram her mind', she explains. 'I get him to give me a few minutes and I picture a nice scenario, romantic scene, erotic movie scene and try to get in the right mindset. I retune my mind. That's the key, the mind', she says, adding that during the day she always flirts and makes eye contact. 'I am suggestive even if I'm not in the mood, because it makes the day harmonious and humorous. We laugh, even during sex. Make it as humorous and light as possible.' She has also helped her mother and sisters get over sexual 'withholding' and begin enjoying sex.

Many women report that they know 'just doing it' can work for them, but they still find it a struggle. Elizabeth (aged thirty-one) from Mount Gambier, South Australia, says:

> When we do have sex it is fun and I am able to reach orgasm easily. I should just do it because we always both feel better after. I just can't understand why when he makes an advance I am so quick to reject. I thought your diary might help to map out these responses.

That's the puzzle. Many women who know that it feels good when they get started are often perplexed by their own reluctance. But much of this stems from this cultural expectation that women shouldn't have sex without desire. 'It goes against the grain of what we've been taught and what we thought we would teach our precious daughters', admits Natalie (aged forty), explaining that the times she's 'just done it' mostly have left her feeling great. 'It's only sex after all', she adds. 'It's great when it's working and not so bad when it's not even working so well. It makes the world go 'round and I'm sure generally a happier place.'

It's only sex after all, she says. It's not as if you are doing something dreadfully painful, or arduous or difficult—like cooking a three-course meal or cleaning years of grit off a filthy oven. There are plenty of women who see it as just part of the give-and-take that makes relationships work. I've had some very funny conversations with women about this bargaining process, which often revolve around cooking! 'You may hate meatballs but you make them because you want to please your husband. It's the same with sex. What's so wrong with that?' asked one woman.

'It's like having to come home and cook when you may not feel like it. It's just something you do sometimes. It's not like a big generous sacrifice. It's like, "Oh, well, why not?"' another told me.

But obviously many women have trouble getting their head into the right space. Georgina (aged twenty-five) from Wagga Wagga, New South Wales, says:

> I feel a lot of pressure to have sex as often as 'expected' if a few days go by. If we have not had sex then I know my husband will be making comments or showing signs of initiation on his part, and honestly I sometimes initiate and have sex just so I don't have him at me and I don't have to feel the pressure. I have this sense of relief after, knowing that there will be a few days before he will be at me again.

She hates the pressure, would love him to back off, but then acknowledges that

> sometimes I think if it wasn't for that pressure I don't know how much sex we would actually have. When we have sex I do very much enjoy it, but it is this head thing. Once we are in the moment it always feels great, the closeness and the love, but it's just that getting there isn't that easy.

No, it isn't always so easy. And that's where the complexities really come in. There are so many factors that interfere with women's 'willingness to be receptive', which, as Rosemary Basson explains, is the essence of the 'just do it' approach.[10] The woman who is resentful about her partner's failure to share the housework; the mother wrung out by catering to the children's needs; the woman partnered by a man who is inconsiderate, mean, nasty, indifferent to her emotional state: Why would they want to be generous? Why would they be receptive?

Antonia (aged fifty-eight) is a busy woman. She works full-time as an office manager in Sydney and then comes home to her second shift, looking after the home she shares with her husband, Angus. She's always up at the crack of dawn, often around 5 a.m., because she likes to get her jobs done before leaving for work.

When her morning chores are finished, she brings her husband a cup of tea, takes off her clothes, gets back into bed and has sex—almost every day.

This is not an easy marriage. 'Sometimes I just love him so much and at other times I want nothing to do with him', she says. 'We seem to get on better during the working week. Each weekend we almost get divorced.' She acknowledges that over the years they have had a lot of conflict, over money, children, housework, sex. 'He is so inconsiderate', she writes:

> He almost never notices things that need to be done around the house that take up my time. He doesn't have much to do and I have heaps to do. I have told him that if he were to help me it would make it easier for me. But when he does do one or two things he expects praise and instant reward.

This woman is happy to have sex every day, but for her husband, that is never enough. Here's a typical diary entry from Antonia:

> We had sex this morning and it was enjoyable as my husband shared a sexual fantasy with me. I used the vibrator to have an orgasm. We went back to sleep for a few hours. I got up to get ready for work. My husband asked me to come back to bed several times. I got annoyed because I had been busy and he did nothing. Got home, brought in washing and started making dinner. Tuna casserole was not as good as usual as I didn't put cheese in the casserole, only on top. I went to bed at 8 p.m. as I was tired. Husband wanted sex but I was too tired. He became cranky and made nasty remarks to me.

Angus often drives Antonia crazy. She's resentful about his constant demands for sex, particularly when he so often seems indifferent to her emotional needs and health issues. Antonia talks about the very active and enjoyable sex life they originally shared together: 'This changed when I realised my husband is determined to have sex no matter how I feel. For instance, if I feel sick and don't feel like sex he ridicules me and makes fun of me. If I say no to sex he often gets mean and nasty'.

I asked her to explain why, in these circumstances, she seems happy to have sex so often. Her answer is touching. 'I feel he is my soul mate', she says, talking about how well he knows her, how comfortable she feels with him. She acknowledges that she is pushed by his expectation that they should have sex often. But there's also her own 'need for physical comfort and pleasure … wanting to feel closer, both physically and mentally'. And when they have sex, she experiences a feeling of peace, a sense that 'it's right'.

There's no question that this woman has a very strong 'willingness to be receptive', but not all the time. The real tension in their relationship is that this accommodating woman simply can't make her husband understand that there are times when, soul mate or no soul mate, she simply doesn't feel like sex: 'Like when I am unwell or tired, annoyed, busy, anxious, under pressure, stressed, distracted or a combination of these feelings'.

And that's the tension that plays out, day after day, in their diaries.

Friday, 28 September 2007—Antonia's diary

I got up early to make breakfast then took my clothes off and went back to bed. Angus said, 'You don't feel like sex, do you?' I said, 'No. I have a pain in my side'. Angus then sulked and said it will be a horrible weekend and he wouldn't go to the coast with me. He also told me how lucky I was that he paid for my car so I could drive to work. I felt annoyed by his attitude. I still had a pain in my side when I came home so went to bed early.

Friday, 28 September 2007—Angus's diary

It was Antonia's early to work day and she made an excuse about the sex and had a shower and went to work. I think she wanted to get out of having sex. It's a pity when she does that as I mentioned before I get hurt and rejected. I need to get over that but I sometimes think if I felt indifferent to her and sex then maybe I would not have a relationship at all. With all the other pressures it is vital to have a sexual relationship with Antonia. I don't think she feels as strongly about it as I do.

They often have great times together. But then he still wants more.

Wednesday, 3 October 2007—Antonia's diary

I took off my clothes and came back to bed and cuddled Angus. I felt tired and didn't feel much like sex. Angus got upset and turned away from me. We were both home that day so later Angus tried to have sex with me in the kitchen but I was not interested and it didn't work. I went out to meet our new grandchild. The baby is so tiny and sweet. Later we went back to bed. I felt more relaxed and the sex felt good and we both enjoyed it. Angus then asked how many times we could have sex today. I felt annoyed because I have other things to do while he does not.

Wednesday, 3 October 2007—Angus's diary

Antonia's day off and all seems well. She came back to bed undressed and we had a lot of cuddles and touching. It's good to cuddle for longer as it makes us closer and I feel intimate with her. She had her legs waxed and visited our new grandson. After lunch she went to have a sleep and I went with her. It wasn't long before she said she would like to do it again. This time she wanted to have sex while she knelt up on the bed with me standing behind her. I penetrated very deeply and it felt very good. That made her feel good and she became quite aroused. I had a fabulous orgasm and she felt very good about my enjoyment. I dressed and she commenced to use her vibrator because she continued to be aroused. We were feeling very close to each other. I cooked tea for her and she enjoyed it. I also cleaned up after tea.

Angus believes that when they do have sex, it brings them closer together, leaves them feeling relaxed and happy. He's eternally frustrated that Antonia can never just forget about all her chores, her worries:

I always like to have sex and it makes me forget the other stuff. Yes, I use sex to escape all sorts of things and I find it the most compelling thing I do. I also like to think that by doing it we keep a strong bond. I can just feel sexually aroused in her presence and I forget all the other pressures. But Antonia can't separate the external influences from her sex desire and desire always loses.

Desire always loses? That simply isn't true. Antonia is a most sexually generous woman, but she still can't get through to him that their emotional connection sets the scene for her desire. 'What I always said to him was fix the relationship and then the sex will be good', she says, reporting that her husband would always say the opposite was true: 'Fix the sex and then the relationship will be good'. The battle continues.

In this complex web of wants and needs, sex is a vital element, a fragile point of connection. Everyone knows that—that sex, good sex, can bring them closer to their partner. That's what makes the 'just do it' idea so attractive. But for women like Phoebe (aged thirty-six) from Melbourne, that still doesn't solve all the problems of maintaining a good sexual relationship. She writes very thoughtfully about the battle which takes place in her mind:

Well the stand-off ended last night, and while I was in a snuggly mood Larry was feeling all passionate. He was 100 per cent and I was at about 25 per cent and in my mind I must admit the concept of 'Why should I do this if I don't really feel like it?' started to play. This is actually very annoying because there is a part of me that wants to have sex and relax and I think feeling put out and like a victim is really damaging to embracing a healthy sex life. I do believe I have been influenced by the idea that I am being taken advantage of if I have sex when I'm not into it. But it isn't just academic—I do feel coerced in some way. What is confusing is [that] Larry is actually expressing passion for me and in some way I am rejecting it—is it a power play?

Phoebe concludes that part of the problem for her is the 'gulf between what I imagine sex to be like and how it really is, and I don't feel that I have the power to make it my way'. She explains she often gets cranky because 'once it gets going he is the one who is all loud and moany and all over me and I start to feel put off—maybe because I am not in control or because it isn't going like I had imagined'. So what does she want?

My way would be more slow, personal and involve looking at each other's faces more and going at my pace and rhythm— rhythm is very important for me to climax. Larry often seems to change pace at the wrong time because he says he can't help it.

But even knowing all that, sometimes she can get past this yearning for the type of sex she really wants and she just does it: 'Last night I was too tired for much and decided to not go into the head stuff and focused on the fact that it is good that my husband is into me (even if it's not specifically the way I would like it to be) and enjoy the cuddle'.

Perhaps the most intriguing response to the 'just do it' idea came from Natalie. She's an Australian woman, now based in

London, who'd read my discussion of the issue on a motherhood website. She wrote about taking 'just do it' to a new level:

> To all you tired mums out there, you'd actually be amazed how many times hubby will say 'Please, no, I am too tired, too busy etc.' if you DO make a move. Those boys are bluffing. They are just like us in so many ways—wanting to feel loved and MAKE LOVE but actually as exhausted as us girls! Give it a go and firstly HE will stop pestering you (being pestered for sex is the biggest turn off for me) and you will realise that having sex can be a fun game for you as a woman.

How to go about this? Natalie had very detailed instructions:

> Hit him when you kiss him at the door ('Hello darling, how about it? Have you got a minute just quickly now?') and when he's leaving for the office in the morning ('That tie looks great but before you put it on, haven't you got time for a few quick minutes to make love to me?') or when you meet him at an office function ('Hello darling. Let's leave early so we can take a hotel room and make love before going home to the baby-sitter!') etc.

She also told me about how she puts this into practice in her relationship:

> The last sex we had was last Wednesday. When we arrived home after an office function I lent across to kiss him as he finished parking the car and said, 'Let's make out'. He was gobsmacked. I undid his fly—this is SO not me but I went for it—and after a second or two I said, 'Come on, let's get home'. The thrill of the 'change of pace' had been so much that he was compliant to the letter and we had such a good time in bed. On Friday before he left I was out of bed first and when I came back from the ensuite to dress I said to him (still in bed), 'How about it, let's go again' … he groaned (a happy groan) and said, 'Please darling! Wednesday almost killed me!'

So her idea was not to just do it when her hubby approached her, but to seize the initiative, again and again:

> I am yet to prove it but I suspect this will mean no MORE sex but he will feel as if he is getting more. His recent mantra has been 'I never get any' but since I've started with sexy come on comments (albeit at deliberately inconvenient moments mostly) he seems happier than ever. Bless the boy!
>
> And for me, I feel it is a victory for me. A bit of control finally. A bit of a say in it too. Because I had shown that I was in fact capable of taking the lead it gave me confidence and got me under the sheets—proving that there is libido there if we just dare turn on the tap! It also helped me feel empowered when I was saying no, that I could raise an eyebrow with some promise to him that something may just be around the corner when he least expected it next.

Natalie is onto something. On its own, 'just do it' won't change very much. But what can really make a difference for women is for them to feel they can be in charge of the action, rather than always being pursued. I talked to some of my female diarists about this, women who were endlessly feeling put-upon. They embarked on a little experiment to see if taking charge made a difference. Here's one response:

> Just to let you know that the 'new me' has started. Came home late last night from a Tupperware party of all things and jumped my husband (my Tupperware parties always include alcohol). It was around 12.30 a.m. and I thought if he did this to me I would be so angry. He wasn't. He was very happy to participate and he thanked me afterwards. Now I just have to keep it up. And it wasn't terrible. I enjoyed it.

The women found they often felt better about sex if they were the ones making the move. But, unlike Natalie's husband, there were plenty of men who showed absolutely no sign of ever having enough, even when their partners came on to them again and again.

Sheri is a 41-year-old mother of three from Mount Isa in Queensland who describes her sexual drive as 'non-existent'. She's stressed out over her husband's constant sexual demands and feels guilty about rejecting him. Her decision to try taking charge was a seismic shift in their relations.

Friday, 19 October 2007—Sheri's diary

Well today I gave it my best. I pounced on my husband first thing this morning when he made overtones about having sex. It terrified me. The kids were in the bathroom right next to our room. My head was telling me to back out and not go through with it, but I stuck with it. We had the proverbial quickie, leaving me about five minutes to get the kids into the car and at school. Amazingly it was very satisfying sex. The look on Alec's face was one of complete amazement. He must think I've finally lost the plot. And I must confess it took me the rest of the morning to get over myself.

Her husband certainly wasn't complaining. Here are his comments about that surprising morning.

Friday, 19 October 2007—Alec's diary

The day started pretty much like any other day with the usual chaos, getting ready for work and school. It was just at the moment when we were ready to leave, when what occurred can only be described as not normal behaviour … in a playful and provocative way, Sheri went for the 'grope' while I walked past her in the kitchen.

It really wasn't more than a quick touch and brush up. I responded with a throwaway comment—'I'm game if you are'—and was already dismissing it in my mind when, much to my surprise and before I knew it, we were in the bedroom with both of us almost ripping at each other's clothing (meanwhile the kids were outside waiting to leave, brushing their teeth etc.). We did it then and there, letting all inhibitions go completely and having what can only be described as a fantastic way to start the working day.

It was frenetic, exciting, powerful, lustful and satisfying, all within the space of less than five minutes. Everything that good satisfying sex should be. I can say with complete honesty that the sexual events of the day were, without doubt, one of the most satisfying and pleasurable I can remember for a very long time.

Yet pretty soon it became obvious that the plan wasn't working. Sheri was exhausted and Alec was simply lapping it up.

Saturday, 20 October 2007—Sheri's diary

I've cornered him in the bathroom, the bedroom, wherever I can find him—jumped him at any given opportunity. He's lovin' it. I feel completely exhausted. And he's not saying no!! Maybe he's afraid the well is going to dry up again or he's just too afraid to say no. Personally I think this is everything he's always dreamed of. I married Mr Insatiable!!

Sunday, 21 October 2007—Sheri's diary

How long do I have to keep this up to get a result? I don't think I'm getting the desired result. I'm starting to wonder what it is that I gain from this exercise. Yes, the sex has been enjoyable, but Alec doesn't seem to be getting tired of it. No, he's not pursuing me for sex, but he really hasn't had to either. There's been more sex in this house in the past few days than there has [been] in the last six months! He's having a great time and I think he'd happily continue on this way for the rest of his life. I need a rest!

So Natalie's plan of wearing men out isn't always a goer. But the issue of agency is an important one. Some women, such as

Natalie, found that seizing the initiative resulted in significant shifts in the dynamics within the relationship:

> Yes, I do believe that if I initiate it, I don't feel that I am being harassed, groped, hassled. And even if I am not totally in the mood (still waiting for that feeling to come back!), it allows me to approach Bill and not feel like an object. When he is doing all the come on I have the walls up before we even begin. There is no chance of me enjoying myself in the slightest.

US author Charla Muller came to the same realisation, but only after taking the extraordinary step of offering her husband, Brad, sex every night for a year as a very special fortieth birthday present. Her book *365 Nights: A Memoir of Intimacy* documents this memorable year, starting with Brad's stunned reaction to her offer of the 'Gift'. 'He was so taken by surprise that he stumbled over our son's fire truck and landed, legs akimbo, in his leather chair', she says.[11]

Her friends were shocked. 'An entire year!' they said to her. 'Why not a week, or a month. It was as if they wanted to slap me about the ear and yell, "What in heaven's name were you think-ing!"' The very suggestion was enough to make them nervous: 'Whatever you do, do *not* tell my husband!' one woman told her.

Muller acknowledges that their sex life was fairly abysmal before she came up with this great idea, since she'd 'made a career out of dodging sex with my nice husband'. It is only when they get in the rhythm of having sex each day and start to talk more freely about their sex lives that she learns how bad it was for her husband. He tells her, 'I know you're avoiding sex and it burns me out. It's humiliating to have to barter for sex … I'm your husband, for Pete's sake, not some cheesy college guy looking to get lucky'.

As the 365 days go by, we learn very little about what actually happens between the couple in the bedroom—Muller's a bible-studying, North Carolina old-school type of woman and very squeamish about revealing personal details. But as a result of doing 'it' every day, she reported that much started to change: 'Brad and I flowed better as a couple. We were happier ... Our house [became] better because we were both more agreeable, more helpful and more solicitous to each other'. She comes to realise that just doing it is serving her well. 'I had spent so much time pre-Gift getting worked up over avoiding sex because the thought of it stressed me out, that I failed to see that going on the offensive would serve me (and Brad) much better', she says, reporting that her daily dose of 'little endorphins pinging around her body' did wonders to help her forget about daily stresses.

But she still finds the going tough, hitting a wall around the tenth month, when we find her talking about the Gift as 'my stupid idea' and 'a hidden cross to bear'. Meanwhile, Brad just loves it. According to Muller: 'Brad is really, really kid-like happy. If you want to see what an adult Disney World would be like, have sex with your husband more often. Brad was practically giddy—only a hat with mouse ears would have made the picture more complete'.

The saddest moment in a surprisingly dull book is when, in the seventh month of the Gift, Brad asks Charla what she wants for her birthday the following month. While she ponders on a day at a spa, he comes up with the cheeky suggestion: 'Well, what about sex for a year?'

'I sat up horrified. "Are you kidding me? How about no sex for a year?" He didn't utter another word, shocked at the vehemence of my reply. The happy, insouciant look on his face was gone', writes Muller.

OK, she's not up for ongoing daily sex—not by a long shot. But the Gift did teach Muller a few things:

> I discovered that despite our busy lives, I *do* have time for quality intimacy on a regular basis. If I can assemble twenty

goody bags for a birthday party, do four loads of laundry, answer a few e-mails, shower, empty the dishwasher, take a conference call and make all the beds before I take my kids to pre-school, I can figure out how to take twenty minutes to get up close and personal with Brad.

Here, too, there's the realisation that desire needn't be an obstacle to regular lovemaking. A year of having sex each day has done nothing to change Charla Muller's basic sexual drive, which is still pretty low. What has changed is her attitude. She's learnt that taking the initiative and having regular sex makes for a closer, more intimate relationship with a far more cheerful husband.

So she's advising women to just do it, but not necessarily every day. Her recommended dose of sex is far less ambitious—twice whatever you are doing now. Just put sex higher up in the to-do list, she says. Women should also stop over-analysing whether they want to, or what's in it for them; sometimes they just need to say *yes*. Here she explains why:

> I married a person with feelings and a sex drive and a desire to connect. I signed on for this so I can't be surprised or resentful [if] Brad wants something, even when it is not at the top of the list. And I not only have to participate, I need to thoughtfully initiate and really mean it.

What's most striking about Muller's memoir is not her meagre reports of their daily sex, but the conversations that strike up between the pair. She learns what it is like to be constantly knocked back. 'It really sucks to get rejected all the time', Brad tells her. You shouldn't take it personally, she responds. 'Why not. I'm your husband! How do you want me to take it?' he replies sharply.[12]

Men do take it very personally. But it is very rare that they'll talk about it. The miracle of the sex diaries was that they opened the door to those feelings and it all just poured out.

6

Juicy Tomatoes and the Celery Stick Men

Joan Sewell always envied lusty women. In an interview about her book *I'd Rather Eat Chocolate: Learning to Love My Low Libido*, Sewell grumbles about her low sex drive and mentions a conversation with a woman who described herself as a juicy tomato. 'If you were a vegetable, what would you be?' the interviewer asked Sewell. 'I don't know, maybe a celery stalk', she replied.[1]

My sex diaries are full of celery sticks. Sadly, most women end up in this end of the vegetable patch. But there *are* juicy tomatoes. There are women who constantly crave sex, who want sex, year in, year out, and end up mighty miserable if it is in short supply.

Anthea's relationship was already teetering when she first started writing for me. The 33-year-old Melbourne woman explained that her partner was a wonderful, caring man, but she had begun to realise they were completely sexually incompatible:

> I am very, very sexually aggressive and experienced. I cannot settle for mediocre sex, no matter how much I try. I have, since I left my ten-year marriage, never been in a monogamous relationship because I have never been sexually sated by only having one partner. My sexual history would be perceived by many as being promiscuous; however, I do not do one night stands or meaningless relationships. I just happen to have,

usually, at least three concurrent sexual partners who all know I am not being monogamous.

Her friends accuse her of acting like a man, by placing too much emphasis on sex:

> But sex is important. It is part of a healthy life. I practise safe sex; I do not put myself in dangerous situations but I choose to have a fulfilled sex life. Right now, sex is too important a part of my life for me to stick with one average partner when I know I can once again be satisfied sexually if I start to go to my lovers again.

The sexual reticence of her nervous, considerate partner was driving her crazy. 'His innocence and inexperience [which] I found slightly cute before now frustrates and infuriates me. I cannot get him to a point where he satisfies me. I can reach orgasm but the sex I crave he is not able to give me', she says. Anthea explains what she is missing:

> The most incredible sex I ever had was a four day fling with an American guy, ten years my junior. From the outset it was aggressive, hard, powerful and incredible, so much so I cannot really begin to do it justice with a description. During our second day together, I gave him my vibrator to do what he chose with. His response was to throw me to the bed, tie me up with a tie that happened to be hanging on my bedroom door and then use the vibrator on me to get me to reach multiple orgasms. He said nothing before we did this, there was no discussion, he took charge, and it was incredible. He was also a trained marine and so there was a great deal of arousal for me, knowing I was with someone who could be so forcefully dominant. Yet I trusted [him] fully because I knew he was very well trained to know his limits as well as those of others.
>
> In stark contrast, after my current partner and I had been together for nearly a month, I used my vibrator on myself while

encouraging him to watch me as part of foreplay. He was so freaked out he went soft and we were unable to continue having sex. The former, not the latter, is the kind of sex I am used to. This is not an isolated incident. He does not know how to initiate sex, and I cannot fathom how that is possible. JUST DO IT! I fear he is so sexually inexperienced and lacking confidence, I will never be able to get him to a level of sexuality that will satisfy me.

I have returned once in the past week to one of my lovers. It was one night of aggressive, all over the room, make a huge mess, knock-stuff-off-tables kind of sex. The kind of sex I crave. I also like slow, gentle sex but there are days when, quite bluntly, I just want to be fucked, and my partner is unable to do that. He tells me he wants to spend the rest of his life with me but sex is too important to me to live my life with mediocre sex. I will not do it.

She's one hell of a juicy tomato. But she has company. Of the ninety-eight couples who took part in my research, ten of the women complained they weren't getting enough sex. It's difficult to know just how common it is for women to be sexually frustrated due to this type of desire discrepancy. The *Sex in Australia* survey, which involved almost twenty thousand people, found that 24 per cent of the men surveyed wanted sex at least daily, compared with 8 per cent of the women.[2] But these figures included men and women of all ages and at varying stages of their relationships, so we have no idea how many in that 8 per cent are genuine juicy tomatoes, remaining lusty throughout their lives.

Of course, there are sexually driven women who aren't missing out because they have met their match—women like Gay (aged thirty-six) from Alice Springs. When she first wrote to me, she had only recently left her husband:

One of the key reasons was that I was sick of always being the one to ask for sex and being told, 'Can't we just sleep?' or being told I put him under too much pressure to perform. My ex-husband had a lower drive than me and I was constantly rejected. I used to even say to him that I couldn't believe here was a 50-year-old man complaining that he was being hassled for sex from someone sixteen years younger than him!

She is now living with Bart, a jockey-sized man with a huge libido, just as large as hers. 'We have moved in together and still are having sex up to three times a day; he is multi-orgasmic and I am having the time of my life', she said first. Nine months later, she reported that the sex had quietened down a little but that they still have it every day, often twice a day.

But with most of my other lusty couples, the women reported that it was the strong male drive that set the hectic pace of their lovemaking. When I suggested to Alice, from Bathurst, that she was one of my juicy tomatoes, she was delighted. 'It sounds so delicious and voluptuous', the fifty-six year old responded happily. Here's a couple who have been married for thirty-four years and are still having sex five or six times a week, sometimes multiple sessions in one day. Yet she says she is interested in having so much sex mainly because her husband, Shane, 'loves it and me so generously. If I was with a partner who wasn't so keen I'm not sure what my interest would be. I wonder how much I would bother about pleasuring a partner who wasn't so interested'. She adds that in those circumstances, she would probably go in for surreptitious self-pleasuring.

Alice tells me she loves being the snake charmer, revelling in her power to attract Shane and have him respond to her advances: 'It is charming and exciting to see how aroused Shane gets and have him pay attention to me'. There are others like her—women who love being wanted, who find that their own libido flourishes due to constant passion and attention from their lovers. And, like Alice, they have no idea how they would respond if they were with a man who didn't want them.

But my diarists also included women living with men who rarely want them—and boy, are they an unhappy bunch. As I mentioned in Chapter 3, four of the ten women with notably stronger drives than their partners ended their relationships during the six to nine months in which they were writing for me. And others, like Sasha (aged forty-four) from Cairns, were thinking long and hard of doing likewise. In her first letter to me, Sasha said she was thinking about leaving her partner of two-and-a-half years 'due to sexual reasons'. This isn't the first time she has run into this problem:

> I am forty-four, slim, long blonde hair and desirable to 'many' men except the one I'm with. Why is this? I have only ever had one sexually compatible relationship in my whole life but he was extremely immature and irresponsible in important areas and that led to the death of that relationship.

And now she's struggling with Vance, who told her he was a 'fucking bronco' when they met but has turned out to be far from it:

> When I met him he claimed to be at the point where he hadn't had sex for so long that he should check in to a monastery. I thought that was kind of 'cute'—a desperately sex starved guy that I actually clicked with. But when it came to doing it he kept on going limp. Reasons—too hot or anxious about perfor-mance failure. So as a means of assisting him in re-igniting his body's responses I regularly gave him oral sex and hand jobs with nothing in return from him. I discovered not too far into the relationship that he didn't like giving me pleasure. By this stage (isn't this always the way?) I was in love with him. Stupid me! Haven't learnt YET. So I resigned myself to the fact that he didn't really have any interest in pleasuring me that much and was more interested in his needs being met. As I had become quite emotionally attached I resigned myself to the fact I would have to get off with intercourse, which I can.

That's what she gets—once every month: 'No actual fore-play, just hop on and off for the same usual once a month horse ride which I will say is FABULOUS. Lasts about ten to fifteen minutes then I wait another month. But I cry these days after sex. It's such a huge release'.

Sasha would have sex every day if she could. And it is not just sex she is missing:

> I am a very tactile person and so not to have much actual touching and affection makes me feel starved. I get tired of being the one to initiate. If I go to him for a cuddle or a kiss it will happen but I'd like him to be the one that wants more than one minute of touch per day.

Vance is avoiding sex with her but he does have an outlet, as Sasha explains:

> The only time he is interested in sex is if I have been out all day and he's been home not working and on the computer, I think. Before I met him he had been on his own for eight years and his contact with women in a sexual sense was porn on the computer. The reason I know he's doing this is because I caught him out one day. How can a guy say he loves you, wait until you leave the house then get onto the computer and drool over untouchable women and then not want sex with you? I am still angry with him for making me believe initially that he enjoyed pleasuring me and he was a 'fucking bronco'. He's the sort of guy you'd think would be 'banging' a chick every day—tall, muscled out, long hair, good looking. But what I truly found was that he hates oral, he gets right into the women on the Net, not me, and lies about it and doesn't like sex if it involves effort on his part. So why do I stay? I want to leave all the time.

She then explains that her children's close relationship with Vance is one reason why she is reluctant to go. Sasha has recently moved to another bedroom, which helps a little, but she's still very unhappy about her situation:

> So what do I do? My gut says stay but go out and root around. I have a lot of 'friends' that would drop everything for me and do everything to please me sexually and there are a couple that are excellent lovers. But it's not them that I'm in love with. I know people in their fifties and sixties who still do it two to three times a week!! That shits me. I work myself most days to exhaustion so my body won't hear the screaming libido. I am hoping that as I get older this dreaded nympho thing subsides, but it has got worse as I've got older!!! I am horny EVERY DAY and what I've noticed is that if I masturbate that feeling does not go away—I could get off ten times and still it's there. I have to avoid television programs where there are love scenes or sex, places where lovey couples go. My self-esteem is shit over this. True, I've got eggs in other baskets, but this is a BIG EGG.

It's a very big egg—and not just for the high-drive women. Even women with little or no interest in sex end up being pretty miserable when they are the ones being rejected. I can just imagine men chortling as they read this, enjoying the thought of women receiving some of their own medicine. It's certainly true that most men learn to deal with rejection—almost always forced into the role of the initiator, they have no choice but to cop it sweet. But it is the fact that women are so rarely on the other side of the fence that makes this experience particularly painful. They never expect not to be wanted.

Since many of them are surrounded by friends whose partners are driving them mad by wanting sex, these women end up feeling there is something wrong with them. 'I can't tell you how many women have told me they feel there is something abnormal about them because they want sex more than their husbands do', writes Michele Weiner Davis in her 2008 book *The Sex-starved*

Wife. She reports that women often end up questioning their desirability:

> 'Are my boobs too small?' 'Have I gained too much weight?' 'Am I doing something that puts him off when we do have sex?' 'Has he lost his attraction to me because he doesn't think I am pretty anymore?' 'Does he think other women are sexier than me?' 'Does he want me to have plastic surgery?'

These are just some of the ways in which women start to question themselves when faced with their partner's constant rejection, says Weiner Davis.[3]

Sarah (aged thirty-five) cheerfully acknowledges that she has zero interest in sex. But the Geelong woman wasn't always like that:

> In the early days (first year or so of our relationship) my husband and I had prolific sex. Twice a day every day. This was before we were married and obviously a honeymoon period. Not surprisingly this began to taper off over the years (we've been together for eight years). In the last few years (before children) we were probably only having sex about once a week. My husband usually was the initiator and usually I said yes even if I didn't feel like it. This is because once we got started I really enjoyed it (I am lucky enough to be able to have orgasms easily). My husband's sex drive used to be high (in that he usually initiated sex). However, I found that over time my libido has become almost non-existent; that is, I rarely think about or want to initiate sex (even though once I get going I enjoy it). It seems easier just to read a book and go to sleep!

When Sarah first wrote to me, she was pregnant for the second time, which meant daily bouts of severe nausea and vomiting. Her constant sickness in the first pregnancy led to a nine-month period of abstinence, which seems to have totally deflated her husband Philip's libido. 'Since then my husband has NEVER initiated sex', she writes. Since then, they have only had sex when Sarah has initiated it:

> That was only because I felt we should rather than because I really wanted to. I have heard that couples who have regular sex are happier, closer and have better relationships. I had to be very persuasive and do most of the work to get my husband in the mood. I find this role reversal very surprising. Needless to say we only have sex a handful of times a year. I have tried to discuss it with my husband several times and he assures me nothing is wrong and he still finds me attractive etc. He reckons he's just stressed at work. I find this shocking and it's a situation I want very much to rectify.

She has no interest in sex but still finds it shocking that her sex life has dwindled to nothing—even a woman with very low sex drive wants to feel wanted by her husband. So what's going on with him? Well, according to Sarah, her husband is a very inhibited man. After her nausea put a halt to their sex life, Philip found it very difficult to re-establish intimacy and approach her once again. Confirming what Sarah had told me, when I interviewed him I found it wasn't easy to get him to open up—talk about pulling teeth! 'If it's not available to you, you just stop thinking about it. It's hard to get back into the swing of it', was all I could get out of him.

That's the problem with the celery stick men, the men who show little interest in sex. They just won't talk about it. When Michele Weiner Davis published her earlier book, *The Sex-starved Marriage*, she went on dozens of talkback radio shows and received hundreds of emails—from low-drive women and their frustrated partners, from high-drive women, from everyone except the men with low libido.[4] Even when the radio announcers invited these men to call, not a peep was heard from them.

Weiner Davis's latest book—*The Sex-starved Wife*—is based on a survey of men's desire published in *Redbook* magazine.

More than one thousand women responded, with a remarkable 60 per cent reporting that they were at least as interested in sex as their husbands. Weiner Davis is now convinced that there are just as many men with low drive as women, although she acknowledges that's not what most of the research is telling us. The incidence of men with low libido rarely shows up as more than 15 per cent in any one study, although Weiner Davis did find one that reported that low desire was more common in men than in women.[5] (The *Sex in Australia* survey found that 25 per cent of men said they lacked interest in sex, but about a quarter of these men were not in a relationship. This compared with 55 per cent of the women reporting low drive.[6])

So is low desire in men just vastly under-reported? Weiner Davis believes so, arguing that the problem is that men just won't talk about it to researchers, and their wives won't admit what's going on because their partner's lack of interest leaves them feeling unattractive and inadequate. Certainly some prominent US therapists, like David Schnarch, are now reporting that they are seeing just as many men with low desire as women. But this may be due to the recent shift in power in relationships, with unhappy wives succeeding in dragging their sexually uninterested partners to therapists while many sexually deprived men just put up and shut up. All of my experience suggests that men with low libido are comparatively rare.

Yet low-drive men are now in the spotlight in the United States. Another recent US book, *He's Just Not Up for It Anymore*, is based on interviews with men who have stopped having sex, and with the female partners of such men—more than four thousand people took part in the survey. It was hardly surprising that the women who were willing to talk about the sexual lack of interest of their partners outnumbered by two to one the men in this situation who were prepared to discuss it. The book's authors, Bob and

Susan Berkowitz, did well to find more than one thousand men who were prepared to complete a survey about why they'd gone off sex.[7]

The authors found that the women were bewildered by their partners' lack of interest, with two-thirds saying they didn't know the reason for it. Many (57 per cent) saw the men as depressed but only a third of the men admitted this was a problem. Just under half the women reported that the men were angry at them, with just as many men admitting that was quite right. Forty per cent of the women felt their partners no longer saw them as physically attractive, while 32 per cent of the men agreed this was a relevant issue.

Very few women identified the men's top-ranking reasons for being uninterested—namely that their partners weren't sexually adventurous enough (68 per cent) and didn't seem to enjoy sex (61 per cent). While it is rare that men totally give up on having sex when they find themselves with sexually reluctant women, there's no question that this takes the edge off many men's sexual interest. The overwhelming message from so many of my male diarists was that they want to be wanted, they want their women to be eager for sex rather than just putting up with it. They are fed up with doing all the work in sex, being made to feel unwelcome, having to beg and grovel for sexual favours from their women and never feeling that sex is a two-way street. 'We men like to feel desirable too. But when our wives never, or almost never initiate sex, or show any initiative in sex, we begin to wonder. It's no good our wives telling us they love us. They must show us', writes Sam from Brisbane. This also rings true for Craig from Cairns:

> Yes, sex can be boring. In the early days with my wife and I, everything was all so very spontaneous and she was often the instigator of it all—which from a guy's perspective is great as it makes you feel like a million bucks that she finds you

so attractive. But as time ticks on you get into the same old routine. (I would always have to give her the expected average of half an hour to an hour massage, after which time we could get it on but of course it didn't last anywhere near as long as you would have liked—too much previous build-up!). Sometimes this routine was so repetitive that it would put me off trying, particularly if I was in the mood for a hot quickie, or I knew she was likely to be so relaxed that I knew she would no longer be interested in sex by the time I had finished massaging (which would happen frequently—I must admit, I do give a mean massage).

The Berkowitz book reports that the majority of the authors' male respondents 'did not seem to be looking for anything out of the mainstream, just a little positive reinforcement'. Their partners' pleasure was a key issue for the men and it bothered them that their lovers did not seem to enjoy sex. 'These guys don't want a silent partner, they want applause. Men tend to be goal-orientated: they like to know their objectives have been reached', wrote the Berkowitzes.[8]

After encountering constant female reticence, the male libido can just disappear, as Anthony (aged forty-seven) from Hobart is discovering. He is surprised this is happening to him:

> I wonder a lot about this. I used to be the perpetually inter-ested one. What was once utterly unthinkable appears to be my reality: sometimes I just couldn't give a f--k any more. For some strange reason, contrary to a history of this type of close and intimate communication with my wife, I find myself unwilling to raise this topic in recent times. It may have something to do with real conflict in my own head about not whether I want IT or not but that I both want IT and don't want IT. I believe there is both a physical urge and a psychological resistance at work here. The latter seems to be connected to the way in which my wife and I initiate a session.

Anthony always saw himself as having a normal, lusty sex drive, and admits he sees it as 'a sort of death' to find himself losing interest. He ponders at length the reasons for this, which appear to be related to his wife Adele's reluctance to ever openly ask for sex:

> The trouble for me seems to be if Adele makes the first move. It is almost always a touch. There is a signature to it and I know what it means. I have a wish to be able to resist that touch. In my mind there's the thought that if I could only pretend I wasn't interested, if only an erection wouldn't betray me, I would have achieved something. Don't ask me what—I just don't know. When I look at this as objectively as I can, it seems the best case of cutting one's nose (or other appendage) off to spite one's face that I've ever encountered. Interestingly, if she persisted and I was 'found out' then I generally caved in and had great sex—although a bit shamefaced to have been caught out putting her through all that. It seems like such self-destructive behaviour. Even while I was 'resisting' I knew I was playing with fire and that this could cause a change in sexual patterns in our relationship that I figured would not be good in the long run.

That's the heart of the problem—her unwillingness to approach him openly. He yearns for her to admit that she wants him,

> to just say she felt like sex and wanted me to do it to (or with) her. I would like to see her wanting sex the way I want her to want it (now there's a selfish, unrealistic thought!). I would really like her to verbalise her sexual thoughts. Over the years I have tried to move towards that point but have been frustrated by her apparent difficulty in finding the words or willingness to share them. Tactile is OK but it's so damned ambiguous. I don't want to imbue her touch with my meaning; I want to know what she's been thinking to want to touch me. I want to know how she wants sex. I want to be inside her head. It

seems to me that I know pretty much all there is to know about her physically and that the 'last frontier' of intimacy is her thoughts. I want that level of intimacy. It's what turns on my own thoughts and thereby my sexuality with her. If it's absent and she's not willing then I don't want to force her but I do feel sad about it and my sexual feeling tends to diminish.

It's not that she constantly rejects him, but after the great intimacy they have shared together, Anthony is frustrated not to know what is going on inside her head when it comes to sex:

> There have been very few occasions when I can recall that Adele has actually said No to sex. But non-verbal clues, yes. There have been times when I wanted it but would find her getting out of bed to get on with the day's chores. When this appeared to be a regular thing I began to feel rejected. I wondered if 'that's it then'—the good times are over? If I allowed the thought to get hold it could have me sinking into depression, quietness, introversion, distance. I tried to be patient—there was always masturbation. After a time I don't feel like pushing for intimacy any more. I reflect from time to time that I just don't feel sexual any more (or at least not as often). When I get depressed over other things, the sexuality issue just pops into my head as just another reason why I shouldn't feel good about life. I just feel sexless. Amazing isn't it? From sexy-to-busting-point all the way to sexless. A lifetime seems too short for such a transition.

And here he is describing a typical sexual encounter between them.

Saturday, 10 November 2007—Anthony's diary

Before I get out of bed I pick up my book for a half-hour of reading. Adele usually wakes before me and she is reading already. She rests her hand on me and from time to time strokes my skin with tiny finger movements. The movements themselves and the places being touched don't carry any overt sexual overtones at all but the persistence of them tells me she probably wants something. Whether it is to please me or to please her I don't know. I don't trust my judgement about that any more. After a while I begin to think about the possibilities—imagining she wants pleasure—[and] I feel a slight sexual response developing. At the same time, thoughts of resentment also build. There is a sense of being manipulated in this.

Adele persists. She treads a narrow path so well—lots of practice, I suppose. She makes no overt sexual move and thereby avoids making the exchange unambiguous, that is with the potential for rejection. I believe she is trying to be courageous—she would have given up otherwise—and I love her for it. I consider the possibilities and think what an idiot I am being. It also occurs to me that my non-responsiveness is cruel to her. I feel wretched. Why am I so mixed up about something that is supposed to be so wonderful? My thoughts go to 'just doing it' and I put my book down and cuddle up to her. I can't see her face but I'd bet anything that she is smiling.

It is extremely rare to find such an articulate, insightful man who is willing to talk about his declining sexual interest. Anthony is a very good illustration of the fact that there are men who are very sensitive to the nuances of their relationships, whose sexual drive isn't simply a testosterone-driven eternal flame but one that flickers and fades when the man feels angry, or rejected, or emotionally estranged from his partner—or, in Anthony's case, is saddened by his wife's lack of openness about her private sexual thoughts and feelings.

But most men who find themselves in this situation pretend it's not happening. They choose to deny their lack of interest, choose not to know. Michele Weiner Davis's survey found that 74 per cent of the women partnered by men with low drive say they try to talk to their men about their sexual divide, but 55 per cent of the men never want to discuss it. A majority (56 per cent) of these women believe that their husbands aren't bothered by their sexual differences at all.[9]

Weiner Davis's *The Sex-starved Wife* comes up with a list of 'libido busters' that are known to undermine men's sex drive. There's body image—yes, men too can feel bad about their bodies and hence lose interest in sex. There's also stress, job loss, depression, grief, midlife crisis, sexual, emotional or physical abuse, confusion about sexual orientation, infidelity and any number of relationship issues that can lead to hostility or distance between the couple. Now add to these physiological matters such as the diseases and medications which impact on libido (see Chapter 14), and other issues like alcoholism and drug abuse, obesity, sleep problems and lack of exercise.

Just as women's libido can suffer as a result of hormonal changes, particularly during menopause, so too can the male drive be affected by a drop in testosterone. One in 200 men suffer from testosterone deficiency—sometimes as a result of genetic disorders, damage to the testicles, or, rarely, a lack of hormones produced by the brain. But the ageing process also affects the levels of this hormone, with some studies showing that one in ten older men have low testosterone. Testosterone levels peak during adolescence and then drop by about a third between the ages of thirty and eighty, although some men do retain high levels all their lives.

Men with low testosterone levels sometimes show other symptoms besides low drive, like mood changes, poor concentration, low energy, reduced muscle strength, osteoporosis and fatigue, as well as problems with erections. When testing reveals the levels are low, testosterone therapy—in the form of injections, implants, oral capsules, skin patches, creams and gel—can make a great difference to libido. This therapy is not advisable for men with certain medical conditions, however, such as prostate cancer and some other prostate diseases.

Among the causes of low libido is another blockbuster—concern about erections. The Berkowitz survey found that 39 per cent of the women interviewed believed their partners had lost interest in sex because of erectile dysfunction (difficulty achieving or maintaining erections), although only 30 per cent of the men admitted this was part of the problem. Often, men's sense of failure when this happens is so profound that they will avoid sexual contact rather than risk exposing themselves to further disappointment. According to the Berkowitzes:

> Many men shut down completely, afraid that kissing and other displays of affection might be misconstrued and lead to embarrassment. It is easier to pretend fatigue or (not necessarily duplicitously) claim anxiety and stress and far less threatening to masturbate and get a release of tension—no erection necessary. Some men shut down so completely that erectile dysfunction inhibits their ability to feel any desire at all.[10]

A poignant letter was recently posted on a website for men recovering from prostate surgery.[11] A man wrote about finally reaching the point where he was able to communicate with his wife about what happened during the time he was impotent: 'I think she was surprised to learn that I had been going through emotional hell because I recognized that I was having some difficulty and I didn't want her to know it, so I compensated in ways which she totally misread'. He cut down on the frequency of sex, hoping he would perform better if he did it less often. 'She was aware of the reduction and her own self-esteem took a beating because she felt she was no longer desirable', he says. As a postscript to the story, the man finally spoke to his family doctor about it and was assured the problem was in his head and he should just relax and everything would get better. 'Then he took my wife aside and suggested she might lose some weight!'

Humph! That was hardly professional behaviour, particularly since the doctor apparently never investigated whether there were physical causes for the man's erectile problems. But was the doctor overstepping the mark in mentioning the wife's weight problem? The weight issue does loom large in the Berkowitzes list of reasons why men go off sex, with over a third of them saying their partner's weight gain was an issue, while 28 per cent of the women also suggested this was part of the story. Michele Weiner Davis tackles this issue head-on. 'Although it might seem unfair, unreasonable, unenlightened or sexist, sexual attraction is a critical part of a sensual sexual relationship', she writes, suggesting this is hard-wired, part of our programming for reproduction. 'So although your husband might really appreciate you for who you are as a person, his zest for you as a lover might disappear if you have changed physically in significant ways.'[12]

Weiner Davis quotes a man who has lost his drive in just this situation:

> In my case it has to do with the fact that my wife now weighs 50 pounds more than when she married me. She'll do many things to rekindle, that is candlelight dinners, bath sessions, Victoria's Secret, books on love tricks, etc.—all that effort and money on something that doesn't matter. Then she can say, 'I've tried everything. He's simply lost interest in me. Boo-hoo'. Well, why not LOSE SOME WEIGHT? Can you imagine the turn-off when someone 50 pounds overweight dons a teddy and/or thong? But I don't dare breathe a word of that or even imply by actions that she weighs 1 ounce more than she did when I married her.[13]

Of course, there are plenty of women who carry extra weight and are still desired by their sexual partners. Remember Gay from Alice Springs, the high-libido woman who has met her match? Gay cheerfully describes herself as 'obese'. At more than 100 kilograms, she is twice the weight of her partner, and has double-E breasts. Yet this is one of my most sexually active couples. 'We just have the best sex life and he loves me dearly', Gay writes, adding that she finds it strange that women put so much emphasis on trying to make themselves look good:

> Go to the gym, wax lips and eyebrows. We will do all that stuff but some find it hard to lay back and receive and give pleasure from a person they want to spend the rest of their lives with??? I don't get it. It makes him/her happy, it brings people closer and it is much more pleasurable than going on a diet and going to the gym.

Gay suggests there needs to be a change of focus in society, away from what looks good to what feels good. I suspect she's right—most men really appreciate a woman who loves sex, even if she does carry some extra kilos.

Yet there were also women who found themselves turned off when their husbands allowed themselves to get out of shape. In her very first letter, Megan (aged thirty-two), from Perth, talks about the fact that her husband, Terry, has 'let himself go'—put on weight, 'allowed himself to age badly'. She's a woman who works hard to keep herself looking attractive and it pays off. She was one of many diarists who ended up sending me photos of themselves and their families, which was a real treat. After corresponding for so many months, you do wonder what people look like!

In Megan's case, the snaps show a very trim but shapely woman who's right to think of herself as a 'real catch'. She's annoyed at her husband's attitude because she feels he just doesn't care about whether she finds him attractive. 'I feel very rejected by

Terry', says this randy woman who longed for a sexually active marriage. They married young—she got pregnant the first time they had sex—and she quickly discovered that her husband wasn't nearly as interested in sex as she was:

> I've always been disappointed that I didn't get to have the bouncing off the walls, going at it like rabbits start to my life as a sexually active human being. I expected luxurious long days spent in bed with a man who was desperately attracted to me, lots of kissing, slow undressing, hours of foreplay leading up to penetration, where we both climaxed, to be repeated six or seven times in one session. I didn't expect this to last, thinking that it would only be at the start of the relationship, but it has never happened at all in the twelve years we have been together. And let's face it, this far in, it's not going to change is it?

When Megan first wrote to me, she reported that she and Terry were having sex about three or four times a month:

> I am unhappy with both the frequency and the quality of the sex. I've always said jokingly and usually in the company of other men, that I see no reason why one couldn't have sex fourteen times a week, once in the morning and once at night. But I guess I would love to be in a relationship where someone wanted me that regularly.

She explains that she's used to making things happen, working out what she wants and then going all out to achieve it:

> I find getting the right amount of sex really infuriating because it necessarily involves another person, and what they do is ultimately beyond my control. I feel a deep sense of personal failure because it's one thing to be able to make things work for you when you don't have to negotiate with anyone, but I don't seem to be able to make things work when it involves another person. I think I deserve to have a good sex life, because, well, why the hell shouldn't I? I suppose this also causes me

significant vexation, because having an uncooperative partner and a not-so-fab sex life really challenges one of my core beliefs, the belief that I can achieve anything.

Megan complains about how sex has become very formulaic:

I do actually get there nearly every time I have sex (as long as I am in the missionary position), so I can't complain about not climaxing. But I think because I do climax very easily, Terry thinks that the sex is good, and therefore doesn't need any work. I cannot talk to him about how dissatisfied I am with the sex. We have never had good communication. Terry takes any complaint I have about one of his behaviours as a criticism of him personally. We had a friend whose wife was so horrible to him about sex—'Hurry up and get it over with'—that he developed problems maintaining an erection. Now if I try to bring up things I am not happy with concerning the sex, Terry says I will give him 'issues'. I don't believe this though. I think it's an excuse because he doesn't want to change.

Here's one of her first diary entries:

Sex with T when we went to bed. It was initiated by him. It was very formulaic. 1) touch breasts 2) finger clit 3) oral sex on me 4) penetration. I didn't come. Mind you, I know I was being a pretty crap partner, and not reciprocating enough. I don't know if this is some self-fulfilling prophecy—I think it will be crap therefore it is crap.

She copes with her frustration by enjoying regular sessions with her vibrator, which she clearly relishes. Here's a typical diary entry:

Ahh. Much better. Got home and T and the kids were out so I seized the opportunity to deal with my frustration. I turned the stereo up loud and got out my vibe and made myself come fifteen times. Not a bad effort for half an hour's work. Grinning like a Cheshire cat!

What was intriguing about this intelligent, assertive woman was her reluctance not only to talk to her husband in detail about how she felt, but to make any suggestions about how to improve their sex life. When I finally persuaded Terry to talk to me, he told me he was the one who usually initiated sex: 'She's always telling me she doesn't get enough but she also doesn't instigate anything. I find that difficult to deal with'. Megan admitted that was right. 'Well, at the start I used to initiate more, but hardly ever any more, not for years really. Now it's almost exclusively all him.'

Michele Weiner Davis found that many high-drive women react this way when they first find themselves rejected. Unlike many high-drive men, who keep coming back for more even in the face of constant rejection, women married to low-desire men initiate sex far less frequently. 'Because women stretch outside their comfort zones to initiate sex, they recoil when their initial advances are met with rejection and become gun shy', says Weiner Davis, reporting that in marriages where the man has low desire, nearly 37 per cent of couples have sex less than once a month. In marriages where women have lower desire, only 20 per cent have sex so infrequently.[14]

After writing for me for some time, Megan finally decided to try to talk to Terry about what was going on, but it didn't go well:

> Yesterday I told him that I wasn't really happy with some aspects of our relationship. I tried to ask him how he felt, and where he thought things had gone wrong. He wasn't really very responsive. He just said he didn't know what I wanted, and then I said, 'But you don't ask me what I want' and 'Haven't you seen that I have been trying to tell you that I'd like things to be different for years?' He did concede that he did know that I wasn't entirely happy. But it was just one-word answers here and there. He said that I made him feel bad but didn't communicate to me why that was. So I just feel terrible, that

it is my selfishness that has been responsible for his feeling bad, that maybe all our problems stem from me wanting too much. And maybe they are. He's really hurt, understandably. I don't think he's going to become the lover I want if he has no confidence. Shit.

Terry wrote to me with his own sad version of their conversation:

This week hasn't been much fun. Megan decided to sit me down for a chat and proceeded to tell me that I was letting myself go and that I was fat and unattractive. She also added that all of these things made it hard for her to climax when she slept with me. I am very hurt by these comments. I have been losing weight and it's not like I'm even fat. Eighty-two kilograms and 5 foot 11. Better than most I'd reckon at thirty-seven. So silly me says I will try harder but I don't know how I will do this. The next day I didn't even want to look at her I was so upset. Later in the day she rang to tell me she loved me and that she was lucky to have me. She says that we have a lot of good things in our relationship and she just wants it to be the relationship she deserves. Now I don't know what to do. I take it from all that that she doesn't want to see me naked let alone sleep with me. The next day she asked me what was wrong and I told her that she had shattered my confidence.

Unsurprisingly, the couple then went through a rather difficult time together, during which attempts at bridging the gap between them often went awry. Their diaries reveal the ongoing tension.

Wednesday, 26 September 2007—Terry's diary

Last night she was drawing on my back. This is unheard of— her touching me like that. So I lay there for a bit and enjoyed it. Then she ran her finger down my side and it tickled so I laughed and she rolled over, so I turned and cuddled her and we were having a good moment together gently stroking each other and cuddling. But then she pushed me away, saying, 'You always reject me!' I protested and said I was enjoying our time together but she had made up her mind. 'No, you rejected me. That's why I don't make a move on you, it hurts me to be rejected.' I tried to say sorry but it fell on deaf ears. So not much sex to be had here at the moment but plenty of negative energy about.

Wednesday, 26 September 2007—Megan's diary

We got into bed, he turned his back to me and I started stroking his back. He said it was nice. Then I tried to reach around to touch his penis and he started being really silly, saying that it tickled. I felt rejected so I pulled away. He then came over to my side of the bed and cuddled me but it was too late. I was lying there thinking mean thoughts about him. Then I said to him, 'Why did you do that? You could tell I was making an effort to initiate sex with you and you knocked me back'. To which he responded, 'What? What? I didn't knock you back'. He didn't make an effort to make moves on me (it probably would have been unsuccessful), and he fell asleep shortly after.

Megan very easily leaps to the conclusion that she is being rejected. She expects Terry not to be interested in sex and interprets any tiny, negative comment as proof of her pessimism. A couple of days later she is still touchy, but at least this time she persists.

Friday, 28 September 2007—Megan's diary

Last night after the kids were in bed, T was watching television half-lying on the couch and I was sitting with him, between his legs, and I started stroking his leg and then I undid his pants and started to give him a head job. He started laughing, saying my nose was cold, and I said, 'Please don't laugh at me when I am trying to turn you on'. He said, 'I wasn't laughing at you, I was just laughing at your nose'. Anyway, I persisted, and then

I undressed, hastily, and climbed on top of him and had sex. I didn't come—I don't come in that position. Then after he came, I asked him to take me from behind, which he did. I enjoyed it but I didn't come (I usually only come in the missionary position). It was nice, but it probably lasted ten minutes from go to whoa. What I would like is a long session, with the television off, with drawn out foreplay, starting fully dressed, slow undressing, exploration of each other's naked bodies, oral sex, missionary position fucking, finishing off with a hard and fast fuck from behind. To be repeated with slight variations several times over in a day. God, I'd just love to be fucked so much that I am forced to say, 'I am sorry, I can't possibly do it again today!'

Michele Weiner Davis devotes much of *The Sex-starved Wife* to helping high-drive women find a way to overcome their pessimism, and to help their lovers find new interest in sex. She warns against being overly critical and constantly talking to the men about what's wrong with them. 'Too many women talk and talk and talk in the hope that someday their words will get through to these guys', she says, advising the women to quit gabbing and instead take action; to think through the times when the man does show more interest and try to re-create what was happening then; to focus on the exceptions—what was he or she doing differently when the sexual relationship was better?—and to work on changing expectations: instead of expecting rejection and looking for signs that he's not interested, act as if you expect him to want sex and enjoy it. Ask yourself, 'How would I handle this situation differently if I was expecting good things to happen?' So if Megan was with a man she expected to be eager for sex, she wouldn't be turned off by a comment about her cold nose. The advice makes sense.[15]

Once again, Weiner Davis is advising couples to 'just do it'. In this book she's talking to the wives of low-drive men, so instead of suggesting to the men that they just do it, she's giving the same advice to their partners—they must get that canoe into the water and start paddling:

> Lots of people with low sexual desire actually enjoy sex once they get started. They may have to clear out the mental clutter and slowly relax, but when they do, they tell me sex is enjoyable … In my experience men are often surprised by how often their bodies respond even if their minds lag behind.[16]

So the woman should initiate, start pleasuring her partner, and his body is likely to respond, even if the urge wasn't there when she first approached him.

But shouldn't the men also be told to do the initiating? Yes, of course, as Weiner Davis makes clear in her more general book on sex-starved marriages. Whoever has the low desire has an obligation to make it happen, she says.[17] And many of my male diarists report doing just that. Craig writes:

> I have had sex with my wife at times when I have really not felt like it or was not finding her attractive (after fights or when I was really tired), because I know how much it would hurt for me to say no. I have only said no to her once and after witnessing the look of hurt and rejection on her face I never did it to her again.

Yet, considering the reluctance of many celery stick men to admit they have a problem, telling them to just do it may well be a lost cause.

Over the months she wrote for me, Megan ended up making progress towards some of the goals suggested by Weiner Davis. She offered to get up early to have morning sex, which Terry prefers—he starts work early and ends up very tired at night. And she started focusing more on what is good in their relationship rather than what is missing. Here she is writing about how relaxed they are with each other:

Last night I ran a bath and invited T to join me. We have a bath together quite regularly. We were in the bath and he let out this great big whopping fart. I rolled my eyes. It was mildly funny, and it reminds me of how comfortable we are with each other. I'm sort of thinking that maybe hot sex and comfort are mutually exclusive? Like one is the equivalent of a really sexy outfit, high heels, stay-up stockings, a tiny G and a push-up bra, and the other is slippers and your old trackies? We are very affectionate, we do cuddle each other a lot and touch each other.

Gradually things started to settle down. By late October, Megan reported they were having sex twice a week and she was starting to feel more optimistic about their sexual relationship.

Tuesday, 16 October 2007—Megan's diary

When we got into bed last night we had a cuddle and he started kissing my neck, shoulders and back some more. I really liked it, but I was holding back because I had my period. We talked about this and then we kissed some more and I sucked on his testes and penis while he gave himself a hand job. It is obvious that he is making an effort. I was surprised by it—pleasantly surprised. It was nice to feel wanted for a change. I even caught myself thinking, 'Hey maybe I could get back into having sex with him'.

A fortnight later, Terry wrote with a notably more positive report.

Sunday, 28 October 2007—Terry's diary

This last couple of weeks Megan was sick so nothing happening. Then I went away with the kids for cubs so again no action. But later in the week Megan jumped on me and that was really cool but she didn't get there because it was all too short and again no foreplay. Then she did it again and that was the same cool fun and all but she didn't get there. Today we had a bit of a romp and some foreplay and she came. Yeah! That was good. It's been a while and I even got some compliments so all in all it was good.

And Megan was clearly starting to appreciate her husband's efforts a little more.

Tuesday, 13 November 2007—Megan's diary

Yesterday afternoon Terry and I were having a cuddle in our bedroom. The kids were playing in another part of the house. He started stroking me gently and kissing my skin softly which was lovely. Then he gave me a little massage, which was great because I had a sore shoulder. The foreplay probably lasted about twenty minutes or so and then we had sex in the spoons position. I didn't come, but it was the best sex we have had in a long time. I was a bit surprised at how much I enjoyed it. I was making an effort not to find anything I didn't like about it.

Eleven months after she started writing for me, Megan reported being happier,

probably more because I have changed things on the inside, rather than because of any external change in my situation. I really try to focus on the positives in my relationship because focusing on what I wasn't getting was causing me misery. I have a great husband who is a wonderful father and he can fix anything. He is a good earner and his job is flexible and he picks up our kids from school every day. He takes care of a good proportion of the general running of the household and family commitments (tonight he is taking the cat to the vet), freeing me up for my own work. And he cooks a mean curry. Even though the sex isn't what I'd like, at the end of the day his little recipe does the job and he makes me come. I know how lucky I am.

And what about just doing it? Megan is thinking hard about what stops her from taking the initiative:

> I feel really vulnerable. I don't want to put myself out there again, to offer myself to Terry once more, only to be rejected. I know I should just push through this fear and assert my sexuality without worry about how he feels about me, but at the moment I am finding the thought of doing this quite terrifying.

But she's working on it: 'Initiating is on my to-do list'.

In her book *Mating in Captivity*, Esther Perel explains that sexual rejection at the hands of the one we love is particularly hurtful because of our emotional dependence on that primary relationship:

> We are less inclined to be erotically adventurous with the person we depend on for so much and whose opinion is paramount. We'd rather edit ourselves, maintaining a tightly negotiated, acceptable, even boring erotic script, than risk injury. It is no surprise that some of us can freely engage in the perils and adventures of sex only when the emotional stakes are lower— when we love less, or more important, when we are less afraid to lose.[18]

Megan's commitment to her marriage to Terry is at the heart of her fear of pushing for more sex. That's why Terry's rejection matters so much to her.

Juicy tomatoes face a very different situation from high-drive men who are trying to inspire reluctant partners. Terry's throwaway line about Megan giving him 'issues' says it all. Men's fragile control over their capricious penis means they may well have real concerns about being man enough to handle a sexually demanding woman. Think of all those jokes about insatiable women—the threat is real to those men who harbour fears about the adequacy of their 'performance'. It would never occur to most women partnered by high-drive men to be concerned about whether they can keep up with him, to agonise over their own 'performance', and to retreat due to concerns that they won't shape up. Michele Weiner Davis is right to suggest that high-drive women need to tread cautiously but not give up—it's possible to light the fire of a sexually reluctant man, but it surely requires a delicate touch.

7
The World's Most Boring Affair

Adam is only thirty-six, a lusty, married man in the prime of his life. But he has had sex only twice in the past six years. The first time was the night he put a ring on his future wife's finger—that very night they managed to conceive their first child. The next and last time was in December 2005, which resulted in the birth of his second daughter.

Adam hadn't really planned on having a second child at that point, but the unexpected offer of sex was too good to refuse: 'At the time it happened I was in a state of shock and was not about to delay things by saying, "Just hold that thought, honey", while I raced to the chemist'. He now expects 'another few years in the wilderness, if not forever'.

Adam finds his sexual frustration hard to handle—'You see, it is a hard place to be and the shower becomes my best friend'. He's tried to talk to his wife about it, many times, with absolutely no response. He's wondered about visiting prostitutes but is reluctant to spend the money: 'I just cannot justify to myself the expenditure. It takes milk from my babies' mouths, if you can understand'. Five months after he first wrote to me—another five months of no sex—matters had come to a head. The couple had a row; he told his wife how he felt and said if nothing changed they would end up divorced. Her response: 'I do not need nor do

I want, or feel it necessary, to share a physical relationship in our marriage'.

The conversation left Adam totally bewildered. 'It put my mind in a spin', he wrote, spelling out his reluctance to end the marriage—he does still love her, and he knows he would lose out through divorce: 'That would mean I am also divorcing my children whom I hold dear to me'. His life is not filled with anger and the couple live together in harmony. However, his wife won't go for counselling. 'She honestly feels I am the one with the problem', he says. Adam ended up telling her that he would 'need to seek girlfriends to satisfy this part of my life I was missing'. She didn't respond. 'So now I take it upon myself to fulfil this in a discreet way', he told me.

Adam's dilemma goes to the heart of the whole discussion of the sex supply. Surely a monogamous marriage or long-term relationship must imply some mutual commitment to satisfying each other's needs, including sexual needs? If that is not part of the deal, if the sex supply breaks down, then fidelity seems a totally unreasonable demand or expectation. The wonder is how rarely we talk about that. We endlessly hear about the shopping list of expectations—particularly from women, in their search for a faithful, committed, caring soul mate. But somehow, sexual needs never figure in the equation.

Adam's decision to seek out extramarital relationships may prove a workable solution. But it is heresy to suggest such a thing. It's become terribly unfashionable to believe that extramarital sex can ever have a role in preserving marriages. We believe in fidelity—survey after survey confirms the modern commitment to sexual exclusivity. In fact, we seem to be becoming even more conservative on this issue. In 1998, 59 per cent of Australians said that extramarital sex was always wrong.[1] Five years later, the *Sex in Australia* study found that more than three-quarters of respondents thought it was wrong to cheat in *any kind of committed relationship*.[2] Adultery always spells disaster for a marriage, or so everybody seems to believe.

That can be true. I've spent many, many hours over the past thirty years listening to people's stories about affairs. I've consoled friends who have just discovered their partner has been unfaithful—I've seen how devastating it can be to suddenly feel like the outsider. In her novel *The House in Paris*, Elizabeth Bowen writes of jealousy as 'feeling alone against smiling enemies'.[3] That's what happens when you discover you have been cuckolded. You thought yourself encased in the security of marriage but the music had stopped, partners had switched and you were dancing alone.

'In any long-term, intimate relationship, there has to be deep knowledge of the other and a profound trust that what one knows is reliable', says sociologist Annette Lawson in her book *Adultery*. The discovery of an affair can mean the end of that profound trust. Lawson talks about 'the destruction of an imagined past' as the marital history is now rewritten.[4]

I remember talking to a friend whose husband was a banker. Oh, he'd never have an affair—he's far too cheap, she announced to her friends. She painted a funny picture of her frugal husband baulking at the costs inherent in seduction—pricey candlelit dinners, illicit lunches in exclusive restaurants, red roses by the dozen. She was so sure she knew him. How dreadful it would be to have that certainty shot to pieces.

A man once told me of the disquieting experience of overhearing his wife talking to her friends, saying, 'If Lindsay was playing around I would know'. Lindsay was and she didn't.

The sex diaries bear witness to the terrible pain that can occur when an affair is discovered, with many couples talking about the impact on their relationships, both past and present. For some it remains an open wound. Shirley (aged forty-seven) from Mildura, for example, has been married for over twenty-five years. She writes that she and her husband have both had affairs in the past: 'It was an awful time and we didn't gain much from it except pain and sorrow'. Her husband, Luke (aged fifty), talks at length about how the affairs changed him:

> She was the first to have an affair. Wifey has never had an orgasm with me. My previous partners were not a problem so I've worked very hard over the years to help her reach orgasm. When I discovered she had been unfaithful this really seemed a slap in the face after all the hard work and research I had put in over many years. So I had an affair too as a vengeance thing. It turned out the woman I had a fling with was the complete opposite of wifey. Completely orgasmic with numbers as high as ten orgasms in a one hour session. So now sex with wifey doesn't hold the appeal it used to. I can grind away for long periods and finish gasping for breath with an aching back, sore knees etc. while thinking about work or something equally as dull to distract me from my own climax. When I finally relent and climax all I get is grief as she was 'so close'. So it's my fault! Wifey blames me for coming too soon. I feel like crap afterwards. Tell me why I'd look forward to more of the same.

The sad thing is that Shirley knows exactly what's going on in his head. He's been daft enough to tell her—one wonders if their marriage can ever recover. Here's a typical, troubled diary entry from her:

> Went to bed sad last night. I don't know what to say or do. I know Luke thinks our sex life is crap. But how do we get over the fact we don't talk about what's happening in our heads or express how we feel or what we want. Too scared of the out-come. He has only ever said he loves me about three times in our whole time together. I'm no better!!! I'm sure he thinks a

lot about the women he had an affair with. The one that came at the drop of a hat. (So he has said.) I can't do that and never have for him. How do I get out of my mind what he said—how can he go back to sausage when he has had crayfish?

And then there's Max from Gladstone. He's sixty-four years old and had a very successful sex life for thirty-five years. The trouble started with his wife's menopause, when she lost interest in sex. They tried HRT, which did little, and then a new treatment—Livial. Well, that was amazingly successful. This hormonal treatment, which combines HRT with testosterone, turned Max's wife into quite a different person. Yet what happened? She became interested in another man and had an affair.

That was two years ago. The affair is over and Max and his wife are still together, but he is shattered. He's seeing a psychiatrist. 'I still have bad moments of panic when I think about the affair', he tells me, adding that it spoiled everything. Max is convinced that it is the Livial that unleashed the wanton woman in his wife. The startled man writes:

> My wife seems very happy about her new-found sensuality. She even had a vaginal reconstruction at huge cost, which is wonderful for both of us. To make love three times a week is fairly expensive as I seem to need Cialis [medication for erectile dysfunction] if we do it too often. Since taking Livial she behaves like a male; that is, she comments about sex like one of the boys from my tennis group. She talks of affairs as if the more the better, whereas she used to be slightly prudish and conventional. She drinks like me, whereas she used to have half a glass of wine, reluctantly. She initiates sex. How many 60-year-old females initiate sex? For forty years I asked her not to wear pants to bed. Now she doesn't wear anything.

She's even having Brazilian waxes, he adds.

Was it really the Livial that changed everything? More likely it was the affair itself—the woman seeing herself in the lustful eyes of her new lover—that caused the disconcerting flourishing of her sexuality. Well, it was disconcerting for him, but one suspects that her sexual rebirth is likely to have done her the world of good.

Luckily, the torment this man is experiencing is not commonplace. Most people don't have affairs—the *Sex in Australia* survey found that just 2.5 per cent of married men had had an affair in the previous year, compared with 1.2 per cent of women.[5] That said, in terms of cumulative figures, a recent *Australian Women's Weekly* survey of almost fifteen thousand women found that one in seven (14 per cent) had had an affair.[6] And the University of New South Wales's Dr Juliet Richters has examined the recent literature and believes that the true figure may even be just a little higher than this.[7]

Most affairs remain undetected—two in three are never discovered, according to US research. But Annette Lawson found that two-thirds of known affairs had actually been admitted to by the husbands and wives in question, often after some evidence of the affair had been discovered. That's the amazing thing. So many people end up confessing to an affair, which strikes me as the ultimate stupidity. Sure, you may believe you are confessing all to preserve honesty in your marriage, or because he/she deserves the truth, but the reality is that this 'telling' business is all about people not having the backbone to live with their guilt. Telling doesn't right the wrong; it adds to it.

Most couples don't talk openly about these issues. They reach conclusions based only on the most minimal conversations between them. The *Sex in Australia* survey found that women (73 per cent) were far more likely to believe they had an agreement with their partner over the issue than men did (57 per cent).[8]

I spoke to one man who puts his trust in a snippet of conversation with his wife: 'We have theoretically discussed it [infidelity] and decided it's not the most important thing in the world'. That's been enough for him to decide it is OK to go ahead and have the occasional discreet affair. For him, the rule in his marriage is clear—'the betrayal comes in getting caught'.

That's the rule for a fair few of my diarists as well. I had women acknowledging they would turn a blind eye to their partner's affairs; they would choose not to know. Some women who know they are being unreasonable in refusing sex or keeping husbands on short rations did admit that an affair might make sense. Here's Monica from Sydney, whose husband, Greg, lives in a bedroom down the hall since they stopped having sex three years ago:

> I don't think I would mind if my husband had an affair(s) but I wouldn't like it if he left me! If we could maintain the status quo of our marriage while he discreetly had an affair it would take away the guilt I carry, but life is never that easy and what woman would want to just screw a married man with no returns? He's a very moral man though so I can't see it ever happening.

Others have actually told their partners to have affairs or pay for sex. 'Yes, it is true. I have suggested he goes and pays for it, which upset him a bit. What is really scary is I don't think I would mind, as long as he wore double condoms', says Fran. Her husband, Julian, doesn't know how to take this: 'She says she wouldn't care but I just don't know if she's joking'.

Of course, I also heard from many women who don't feel this way, women who see honesty as critical to their marriages. We live in a society which places supreme value on openness and communication in a marriage. 'Affairs really aren't about sex: They are about betrayal', says Shirley Glass, a US extramarital sex guru.[9] The US view is that affairs are an affront to the shared value of openness—philandering is regarded as extremely serious, a symptom of a deeply flawed marriage.

Pamela Druckerman, in her book *Lust in Translation*, points out that of all the peoples in the world, Americans are among the most neurotic about adultery. She suggests that while in many other countries it is seen as a regrettable lapse but not necessarily an unforgivable act of heinous betrayal, adultery crises in America last longer and seem to inflict more emotional torture than in most other places. Australia is heading down the same path, with infidelity now seen as a very serious issue.[10]

'For me, an affair is a deal breaker', writes Lucy (aged thirty-eight) from Sydney. She has talked about the issue with her husband, Noel. 'He knows this and so any move towards an affair on his behalf would mean to me that he's looking for an excuse to end an already struggling relationship.' Yet, given her current indifference to sex and their endless fights about it, she does worry that he might stray. 'I do feel for him, wanting sex more and me not being receptive. I know how urgent and frequent his sex drive is. It does make me worry he'll look elsewhere for what he needs', she says, adding that her husband is very attractive, good looking and charismatic—'Opportunity surrounds him at every turn'.

But it was also clear that there are women who are determined not to address the issue. I had the most fascinating exchange with an expat Aussie, now working as an executive in Japan. Fifty-year-old Norman has been married for eighteen years:

> I love my wife (almost fanatically), we cuddle, do everything together, we are happy just to be with each other. But I am the one who wants sex, and she refuses it. We have had sex six times in the last year. That is a decline from ten the year before. How do I know? Because five years ago I started putting

little stars in my calendar each time. Whenever I raised the topic in the past, she refused to talk about it, point blank. If I suggested a therapist, she would just get angry and fume for a few days. I tried all that in the past, and several other tactics to either activate her, or help her understand my need/want/desire/lust—all to no avail.

Then he found a solution: 'Years ago, I decided that to keep myself sane I would seek enjoyment elsewhere. It has worked'. Norman has had a series of love affairs over the past twenty years. They are never casual flings:

> I do not have casual sex … All my lovers are just that. They are lovers. Each of my partners other than wife have been lovers, not mere bodies to stimulate my desire. Long term relationships. At this point in time I have two girls I see regularly, at least once per week. Have been seeing one of them for nearly three years and the other just on a year now. I have a total of nine girls I could call, arrange a meeting, and they would be willing for us to go to bed the moment we meet. More that are 'maybes'. Girls that have been lovers in the past, but I haven't seen for a while, and whose circumstances may have changed. The length of time I have known them varies, but most over a year, and some for up to fourteen years. Mostly they have always been married—and still are. Our lives remain separate and uncomplicated, yet when together we make love. Sometimes we enter a room, tear at each other's clothes and end up leaning on a wall, sink, or whatever serves as support at the time but it ends with gentle cuddles and caressing on a bed. Often spend nights together, or whole days, warm in each other's arms.
>
> To make love to three different girls in a week is not uncommon. They all know I am married. They all know that we will go home separately. They all accept it, or it doesn't work. Have I lost any? Yes. Some, usually the single ones, tell me they need something more, they want me when they want me,

not when I am available. Totally understandable. It hurts to let them go but I never beg them to stay, as I know I cannot offer and will not pretend to offer a future at this stage. Who knows, maybe one day my circumstances may change and so be it. But now, I love my wife more than anything else.

I have never led a girl astray by telling her I was single; I have always stated my case as it really is. I have met many wonderful women, single, married and from all walks of life. I have found women with the opposite problem to me and our arrangement has been supreme. The fact that I can now sit at home without feeling aggressive because I have that knot demanding untying, makes us a much happier couple. No, she doesn't know. I have an excellent sex life. But not with my wife. I just wish I could get her to share the enjoyment, but I think she has almost completely lost her drive.

His long executive working hours, including weekends and late evenings, make it possible for him to find time for this other life:

Whenever I get a break, when I know I can tweak my schedule (like yesterday), I will take some time to enjoy a lovely encounter with a girlfriend. Yesterday I took the whole day off and spent it in bed, in the arms of a girlfriend. Rented a room, made love, had a bath, made love, ate lunch, went back to bed and watched a DVD then made love again, showered and went home and sat on the sofa watching TV with my wife nestled into me.

His life is neatly divided between his comfortable domestic life with his beloved wife and his restless erotic adventures. It's worked well for many years—for him and for his wife, whether or not she senses it. Affairs are sometimes 'acts of resistance', writes Esther Perel, who is one of the very few therapists willing to acknowledge that affairs can sometimes enhance the primary relationship: 'An illicit liaison can be catastrophic but it can also be a liberation, a source of strength, a healing. Frequently it is all these things at once'. Perel takes issue with the US model of intimate love that celebrates transparency … having no secrets, telling no lies, sharing everything. 'In other cultures, respect is more likely to be expressed with gentle untruths that aim at preserving the partner's honour', she says, arguing that concealment not only maintains marital harmony but is a mark of respect.[11]

There is no question that Norman loves and respects his wife. Driven outside his marriage to satisfy his sexual needs, he now revels in the variety, which spurs him into other erotic adventures. He explains:

> Each person has a different smell, taste, size, shape, urge, rhythm, surge, sound. Some lie in wait, some rise and receive, some reach and take. Some are urgent while others are languid. It is the variety that excites. Would I be able to live with the same style? And perhaps this is why I can still enjoy being at home. Each new girl brings me something new, it may only be subtle, it may be spectacular. Then I take that home, keeping me in perpetual flux, changing and developing. Perhaps my wife sees it? Feels it? Perhaps it is why she is still happy in my arms.

Even the mildest flirtations can sometimes provide that lift —the sexy chat with a work colleague in the lift, intimate details shared with a stranger you sit next to on a flight. They offer a frisson, an erotic charge which we can use to enhance a relationship.

Dan from Brisbane writes to tell me about picking up his four year old from day care:

> It was a cold day and another mother had put on a figure-clinging pair of tights. I nearly fell out of my car when I saw her. It so happened this lady had a child in the same room as my little guy. I tried to look away and play with my son, Josh,

for longer than normal to avoid having to follow this mother to her car. As luck would have it she must have had trouble getting her child into the car as I received another eyeful as she got into her car. She then drove away. I dreamily walked Josh over to my car. He stopped, looked at me and then asked, 'Daddy, why do you have that funny look on your face?' Doh! Yes, you may well ask, son.

When he got home, he told his wife, Susan, about what had happened: 'She could not stop laughing. Later I was putting Josh to bed and Susan took great delight in putting another funny look on my face. Needless to say Josh received a short bedtime story'.

Ester Perel plays with this idea in her book *Mating in Captivity*, suggesting that the menace of the 'third' is intrinsic to the experience of love—the shadow of the third cements the dyad. She most beautifully captures the way in which acknowledging the third can validate the erotic separateness of our partner:

> I know you look at others but I can't fully know what you see. I know others are looking at you but I don't really know who it is they're seeing. Suddenly you're no longer familiar. You're no longer a known entity that I need not bother being curious about. In fact, you're quite a mystery. And I am a little unnerved. Who are you? I want you.[12]

'Who are you? I want you.' That jolt, that sensation of looking at this familiar person through new eyes. My diarists write about this. They are stunned when the discovery of a partner's affair provides an erotic charge. 'To my surprise, instead of feeling angry or upset, I found this a turn on', said Margaret, who discovered that her husband had had a fling early in their marriage.

Hans (aged fifty-nine) tells a similar story. The Sydney man was in his early twenties when he married and was constantly,

Open Marriage and Other Swinging Adventures

Extramarital sex does not always involve deception. That came through loud and clear from the sprinkling of diarists who have open marriages/partnerships. 'Don't just write about affairs', Gay from Alice Springs pleaded with me:

> Most people see an 'affair' as an attraction between two people behind the backs of their partners, but there is no need to lie about sexual relations if you are open with each other. The essence of swinging is the openness and honesty. It is not always successful, but then again, neither is monogamy.

Gay writes about a married friend with a successful open relationship. The woman always has a boyfriend:

> Her husband urges her to find a new boyfriend as he finds her happier if she is getting extra sex and friendship; it's like a hobby. And he also gets sexual benefits from her increased drive. The key is that he knows the men, often meets them. It is an open marriage.

Yet Gay acknowledges it was swinging that led to the end of her own marriage. When she had been married for only a year, she discovered that her husband was seeing prostitutes:

> I was pretty devastated. He could have whatever he wanted with me and didn't want it. It was this discovery that led me to decide to have an open relationship sexually as I had done with partners in the past. Well, this unleashed a beast. The first time he had a threesome with another woman and me he managed to come five times. He had never done that before; he loved it. However, it eventually took over our life and it turned out that all his fantasies were being played out with other people and not me. He would meet them on the internet and on swingers' sites and spend hours on the computer and then he was tired and would go to bed. He spent so much time organising our sex life that we ended up not having one. We had threesomes, foursomes and moresomes, he had three women at once and I had three men at once. We had group parties in our house with up to sixteen people at one time. It became rather bizarre at times.

While their swinging life flourished, at home, sex dwindled to a weekly event:

> He actually told me once that he could only come once a day or it was just all too much for him. Basically this meant that if he was going to see another woman on any given day, I could not have

sex with him. I told him time and time again that swinging is supposed to enhance the home sex life, not hinder it. Meanwhile, he was enjoying having a string of women. We also had couples that we both played with and both of us swapped at the same time.

The end of the marriage came when she discovered he was constantly lying to her about his swinging activities. 'It was obvious that he got off on the secrecy of it all. This caused the major rift and, combined with the lack of sex I was getting from him, instigated the end of our marriage', Gay writes. Yet she still firmly believes these open relationships can work well and enjoys the occasional threesome involving her current partner, Bart, and another woman, or sex with another couple.

The internet has led to a boom in swinging—it's up by 20 to 30 per cent from ten years ago. 'Paul', who runs *Vixsin*, a national swinging magazine, and an associated website (www.vixen.com.au), estimates that 100 000 people in Australia are involved in swinging activities. Gone are the days when swingers were forced to skulk around adult bookshops looking for magazines, and then use snail mail to try to arrange a connection. 'Now it's quite possible for you to post an ad at 5 p.m., have a horde of responses by 6 p.m. and be naked with someone by 9 p.m.',

says Paul, who, with his wife, runs swingers' parties in Melbourne, which remain popular despite the large numbers now meeting privately through the Net.

It was a chance remark to her husband, Alan, that lead Gillian, an Adelaide diarist in her early forties, to embark on her recent swinging adventure. She'd met a man she found attractive and told Alan that she'd found herself fantasising about sex with the guy. She says:

> That opened the whole can of worms when he realised I was serious but would not go out and just do it as of course it would hurt him. It turned out … that he would be perfectly happy for me to do it as long as he knew about it and was there etc. So I looked up the internet. Ah Google! I got many hits. Some of the parties just appeared to be sleazy pick-up joints in rundown bars. One had the word 'upmarket' in it and that tweaked my interest. Anyway, I went to their website and got all the information and showed Alan. He was interested in the parties and we filled in the online application, sent a text to a mobile number, and received the address. And for $70 we gained entrance to a house used only for parties of various kinds.

Gillian reports that it took a while for things to get going:

It was amazing just how open some of the people are. But the vast majority seem to hide behind their drinks and clothes. The parties start at 8.30 p.m., but no one seems to hit the sack until close to 12. I love to flirt, but again, no one seemed to have the courage to do anything until they have had a few drinks under their belt. It may be just because it's Adelaide but I'm unsure of how many actually got laid. I had sex with a rather charismatic man the first night. Alan watched. At one point I was on my knees sucking Alan and being fucked from behind by X. And while I was certainly turned on, it wasn't until X left the room and Alan and I played that I truly let go and orgasmed. I assume I was nervous as Alan was in the room. We went a few weeks later and a lovely lady wanted to be the first to make love to me. It was awesome (although why do woman think they need to move their tongues so quickly —what about languidly building up?) but her husband just wanted to watch. This meant that Alan was not able to join in and boy, would he have loved to fuck her. But again, afterwards we had the time of our lives together.

There were also older diarists who'd experimented with swinging in the past but moved on.

These erotic adventures work well for some people. But while some find they enhance a relationship, other couples come unstuck when new attachments create a hornet's nest of jealousy and emotional upheaval. Open marriage is not for the faint of heart.

relentlessly randy: 'The first few years seemed to consist of regular arguments about my wanting it more than she did. I lost count of the number of early mornings when I would snuggle up with a rampant erection, only to be rebuffed with a "but we did it last night"'. Gradually their sexual relationship improved, he learnt more about pleasing her, but the sexual imbalance remained. Hans ended up having a number of liaisons on trips away over many years—'something I am not proud of', he adds, but notes that he's grateful for what the women taught him because he believes it made him a better lover at home. But the really interesting twist to the story was that, somehow, his wife always found out:

> In the quiet intimacy of pillow talk during foreplay, when she confronted me with a question about something happening on the last trip, I was seldom able to lie to her or deny it. This never seemed to impact adversely on our relationship and, perversely, almost seemed to be a turn on for her. Before we knew it, we'd be going at it hammer and tong.

Looking back, Hans now feels she knew that none of these incidents posed a threat to their marriage. 'I think she may have been quietly grateful to these sisters for accommodating my demands when she couldn't.'

Rosemary thinks her husband might feel the same, if he actually knew she was having an affair. This sexy 35-year-old Sydney woman has been married for eight years to Jeffrey, a man who is far less interested in sex than she is. He's told her a few times that he wouldn't mind if she was unfaithful, and she's convinced that their marriage has improved since she decided to branch out. The lively, intelligent mother of two says:

> Feeling that my husband wasn't completely and solely responsible for my sexual needs made me a lot less resentful of him, and consequently I was nicer to him, complained less and put less pressure on him. He was happier and I was happier. I came to see having a lover as an important part of making my marriage work. It's not the conventional wisdom on how to have a great marriage but I think it works for me.

She adds that she may not always hold this view, 'especially if it ever got out and was a big mess'.

In a wonderful note of irony, Rosemary describes her illicit liaison as the 'World's Most Boring Affair', detailing the endless problems she and her lover have getting together. They met in their workplace and it started off with flirtation, stolen kisses, dirty emails, phone calls and what she calls 'office romping'—

oral sex in each other's offices. But gradually she realised he was stalling about finding the time for a proper sex session. The man had performance anxiety. 'That wasn't doing much for my self-esteem—both my partners not interested in having sex with me!' she wrote. It took her a year to get him into a bedroom and that first time wasn't great:

> He wasn't really hard, and he sort of just mushed it in there and pressed against my pelvis. I didn't really get into it. At one stage, he said, 'You didn't really like that, did you?' I said, 'I didn't not like it'. 'That's the same thing', he responded.

After nearly three years, they have only had four sessions that have included intercourse. Rosemary actually climaxes far more easily with her husband because she needs penetration, which rarely happens with her lover. Despite this, she just loves the extramarital sessions: 'I love the attention he gives me, and the foreplay. I love the way he will go down on me for ages and ages'.

Rosemary is astute enough to realise 'that it is the not having that makes the occasionally having so delicious'. Sex with her lover is glamorous, she writes.

> I realise that it is only glamorous because we don't live together —the familiarity that you establish living with someone eats away at the sexiness of your interactions. If I lived with him and had to listen to him fart, or watch him snore in front of the television, that would make him more ordinary, and probably less sexy to me. I recognise that the reason things seem to be going OK with my lover, Eddie, is that I only want one thing from him, but that if I asked for more we would probably have other issues.

The glamour of the affair contrasts with the comfort and familiarity she shares with her husband—she thinks he is a great dad, that they have a good life together and enjoy each other's company:

> So many things just work well between us. It's just the sex and communication thing where we fall down. I appreciate that I can be myself [around] Jeffrey more than I am around Eddie, but I don't think that familiarity helps our sex life, or our desire for one another.

There's such a build-up to her sessions with Eddie. She plans them long in advance, thinks about what she will wear, what will happen. Here, she's writing about one of their very rare sessions together at a hotel:

> Went up to the room and spent a long time kissing fully dressed on the bed. Then he said, 'You always dress so beautifully, it's almost a shame to have to get you naked'. He began to undress me slowly, touching each bit of skin as it was revealed. 'I'm going to spend a long time admiring you', he said. I undid his shirt and ran my fingers across his chest. That drives him wild. I love feeling so sexy, being able to turn him on with such a small gesture. I kissed his chest, his nipples and his underarms. He has a little patch of hair in the middle of his chest and I love running my tongue through it. After running his fingers around the edge of my bra, he undid it and took it off. He spent a long time kissing my breasts, which was a real turn on for me. Then he removed my G and fingered me delicately. Mmmmm. The foreplay probably lasted about an hour, and then he rolled me on my back. I reached down and got him hard with my hands and then we had intercourse in the missionary position. I came while he was fucking me. Mmmmmm. Fucking awesome. Then we rested, and I stroked his body while he slept a little. I loved just lying with him, being able to be intimate with each other, because it's such a novelty. Then we shared a bath, which was lovely. I was lying between his legs, with my back on his chest,

and he was stroking my breasts and gently teasing my nipples. We returned to the bed and spent more time exploring each other's bodies. I went down on him. I love giving him head. We had sex once more, with him taking me from behind. I didn't come, but I loved it. Then we lay together for a little longer, but then I had to go. I think we were together for about four hours.

Rosemary knows this indulgent session was special because they were away from all the distractions of work and home life:

Jeffrey and I are always trying to carve out a few minutes here and there to have sex but I have taken Jeffrey to hotels before, and it's not the same. We do it quickly (the same way we do at home), and then it's over and he puts on the telly. It's just like being at home, but probably a bit more boring because I can't go off and read a book or check my emails while he is watching crap TV.

While she jokes about living as 'a dirty rotten adulteress', Rosemary still believes it makes for greater happiness for them all:

I'm torn between wanting to get it all from the one relationship and accepting that it's not possible. I thought that the affair would be the easy option—but let me tell you, it's not easy at all! I have to work really hard trying to accept all the external limitations. But I've decided to just accept the way it is because it's worth all the frustration for a few stolen minutes to be in-timate with someone who really digs me sexually.

David Buss and his colleagues at the University of Texas, who are important researchers in this area, have found that one of the major factors motivating women to have affairs is being in an unsatisfying sexual relationship or partnered by men who are un-willing to have regular sex with them. Men are likely to respond similarly, but there's little research on this link, says Buss.[13]

For many women, however, sex is the least of it. There is a substantial body of research showing that unfaithful women are often more interested in an emotional connection rather than a sexual one. Canberra woman Alison (aged fifty-two) was married with three children when she fell for Steve, whom she met while doing a computer course. This extramarital relationship lasted over twenty years. 'I look back on this other relationship with gratitude and no regrets. It was a joy to be in love and to share my life with someone I admired so much and loved to be with', she writes, adding she is enormously thankful that her husband, Oliver, never found out about it.

She now has an extremely close, loving relationship with her husband—they have been together for over forty years. But she was attracted to her lover at the time because he was so different from her husband: 'He was someone who constantly took risks, who wasn't dependent on me for his happiness and appreciated the risky, open me. With Oliver I always kept my enthusiasms and misgivings in check, as he found them threatening'.

This was not a woman who was dissatisfied with her sex life at home—her husband worked hard to keep her happy. Perhaps he worked too hard:

> For Steve and I, sex was a natural extension of an appreciation of each other—sexual activity came out of our sharing of ideas, experiences and being close. But sex was generally at the forefront of Oliver's mind so that rather than wanting to seduce him when I was with him, I would downplay my attractions. On the other hand, I enjoyed seducing Steve. He was easily satisfied, while Oliver always seemed to want more, wanting his pleasure prolonged beyond my interest level. He also worked conscientiously at giving me more pleasure than I really wanted. I wasn't that interested! My pleasures came with the mutual appreciation and in the cuddles and the stillness more than in the rubbing and stroking with the possibility of an orgasm.

She never did climax with Steve. But when she met him, Alison became interested in sex for the first time since being married:

> My body came alive. I felt totally appreciated and my body wanted to respond and give, not only to Steve but also to Oliver. I admit that when I was with Oliver I usually imagined I was with Steve, but this brought out the best in Oliver. He loved my greater interest in sex, my coming alive. He felt wanted and appreciated.

Having always thought of herself as an honest woman, Alison was surprised to find she was able to live for over twenty years with the deceit:

> I felt no guilt about the relationship, the deception or the lies. This love I had, I characterised as 'golden' and to be embraced. On later reflection the relationship was possible because neither of us saw the new relationship as our primary one. Our families took precedence and neither of us wanted or asked for more than we were able to give in time or in how we expressed our love for each other. Of course, the hidden nature of it added to the excitement and generated its own energy.

Eventually that faded; her admiration for her lover disappeared. They still meet for coffee occasionally, but she is no longer hungry for his company or his body.

Reading these stories, what comes through is the power of an affair to elevate ordinary lives to the extraordinary. Yet this is a danger zone for marriages and carries a mighty risk. Among all my diarists, the person who worried me most was Sally. Where other diarists happily shared so many details of their lives—names, phone numbers, even photos of their children—Sally never told me her surname. She is skating on thin ice and mighty nervous— with good reason.

The forty-two year old lives in a small Queensland country town. Her children are now grown up and, after staying home to raise them while doing heaps of volunteer work ('always doing for everyone else'), she's yearning for a life. Sally tells me she became bored, fed up with her life, her reliable, solid husband, her marriage: 'Basically happily married but all very predictable and boring and safe. Hubby hurtling headlong into middle age and I am looking for what I didn't do in my twenties'.

So she has put herself on MySpace, chats online to various men, and takes herself off to local pubs to hear live music. In her first letter, the raunchy woman writes:

> I'm a bit of a legend now, old girl game enough to go out alone and dance with anyone and everyone. Even my hubby puts up with it because now I am a bit of a hotty in bed. I have numerous suitors and I find that a lot of things with three legs are very desirable.

Over the next four months, Sally sends long, detailed diaries about her adventures—the nights out dancing in pubs, flirting with men, and then home to Trev. 'Whenever I get home at 3 a.m. he is soon awake and looking for some action because he naturally assumes I will be hot to trot after my night out. He is VERY predictable', she says. She is indeed hot to trot, and Trev is reaping the rewards from her late-night adventures. Here's a typical diary entry:

> I got home last night at 2.30 a.m., had a quick shower. It was still hot outside and I had been dancing so was very sweaty. I got straight into bed naked and initiated proceedings with Trev. How could I not, after having been around F, C and N all within the space of a few hours? We had good sex: I had a good orgasm and Trev did too. We indulged again this morn-ing with similar success even though we had limited time.

We certainly have a sex life worth reminiscing about now, all due to the changes within me. We both feel a lot more loving towards each other in the first hour or two afterwards but once we start getting on with the daytime drudgery, I just want him to disappear, to leave me to my own little world. I guess I am being very selfish, but I feel entitled to it these days. I feel like I am just using him for sex and to provide me with food and shelter. He probably feels like he is being used at times but he has the hot new me to distract him, I hope.

Her everyday life, however, is still tedious—cooking for adult sons home from university during the holidays, caring for elderly parents, sharing a cuppa with her hubby. Here she describes a day with Trev:

Sunday was another run-of-the-mill Sunday. I suggested we go to movies in afternoon—I am trying to make an effort here. Went to see a dumb comedy that I thought he would like and he suggested we get a gelato afterwards. I didn't really want to but agreed to keep him happy. Another non-event, just sitting there like an old couple, eating in silence.

It's her secret life that makes it all bearable: flirting on email, text messaging, stolen kisses after nights out in the pub, and then, finally, a hot night with one of her internet friends:

During the evening … I kept my distance from G but whenever we looked at each other across the room, it was just electric. It's a wonder people couldn't see the sparks flying between us. We both knew what was to come later … We started touching and kissing and it was just so wonderful. I had no inhibitions at all. I was totally comfortable with this man who I had only met via email three months prior. We spent about an hour in bed getting to know each other's bodies and then he asked if I wanted him to lick my pussy …

And so it went on, the long detailed description of an experience this woman relives again and again. Months later, she writes:

> I still smile to myself when I think of that night in Sydney, all of it, not just the time in motel room. The hours before were electric as well, looks across the room, then standing together, then touching in the taxi, the anticipation all the time, the unknown, not even knowing for sure where it would lead.

For Sally it was a magical night, but then came the soul-searching:

> So what's going on with me? First time I have ever had sex with anyone other than my husband, and I liked it, it felt right. I care about my husband; he has done nothing wrong: nice, safe, dependable man. I am the bad one here. Now that I have done it once with someone else and it felt right, not sure that I trust myself. Am I going to turn into a loose woman? This is not ME. Good, safe Catholic girl gone bad.

There have been scary moments: her married lover in a panic because he fears his wife has discovered his emails to Sally; a young suitor suddenly draws away because he fears it is getting out of control. She gets nervous. In a dark moment, she writes:

> So I guess I am officially a bit of a trollop as a wife. Kissed two other men and had a hot night in bed with a third. I am on a slide I can't get off, I think. What is the official definition of a slut? Several one-night stands would put me in that category, I imagine. Word would get around and that would be the end of me. All I'm going to end up doing is to hurt everyone.

Yet, she continues to enjoy a very active sex life with Trev, though handicapped somewhat by his erection problems:

We did have sex last night. I had a much needed orgasm by usual means, but when Trev resurfaced and tried to get in— nothing. A little, soggy cocktail frankfurt. Don't worry, he still tried to shove it in but I didn't encourage this, so end of story for him. While he was chowing down on me, I didn't know whether to think about G, who has done the real thing, or R, who might well be next. I have to make sure I keep my mouth firmly closed in case I let a name slip out.

It's so sad reading about Trev. Over the months Sally writes for me, there are signs he's becoming tense and anxious.

Saturday, 10 November 2007—Sally's diary

This morning he got up and got dressed and came around my side of the bed and gave me a little kiss and said, 'I love you'. I said, 'I hear that a lot lately'. He wondered why he said it so often. I know why, and he voiced my thoughts exactly: 'Must be my age or my insecurity'. I agreed with him. Was only a light-hearted exchange but hit the nail on the head.

Sunday, 25 November 2007

I went to bed as soon as I finished, just behind Trev. He was really weird, like he hated me. He did give me a small kiss and said, 'See you tomorrow if you are still here'. He is definitely acting more distant towards me, which is fair enough, just giving back as good as he gets I suppose. I almost feel like he is trying out the old saying with me—'Give her enough rope and she'll hang herself'. It seems like he is letting me do what I want and is waiting to see what mess I get myself into.

Monday, 26 November 2007

This morning he got up and got ready for work, completely ignoring me. He said goodbye and didn't kiss me. He always does if I am awake, even if I am in a bad mood. It was really very scary. I don't know if he has seen or heard something he shouldn't have or has put two and two together and come up with .... 100. Wonder if I will ever know. I wasn't game enough to ask what was wrong with him. I had an awful thought that maybe G's wife knew something and had found us and rung and told him to tell his wife to keep away from her husband. Now I am imagining things. Maybe I should just keep to myself and forget about all of them.

By January, however, things seemed to have settled down.

Tuesday, 8 January 2008

We did it again Monday morning. Very, very nice, I was close to having some sort of orgasm without oral but Trev went in for the kill and off I went again. I told Trev he was 'quite good'. He said, 'You are better than brilliant ... can't find a word'. I am feeling quite benevolent towards him at the moment. I am not going to use the word 'love', but I definitely need him, or at least someone, these days.

Saturday, 19 January 2008

Funny thing. Last night Trev tried for a bit but couldn't get it going. I wasn't in the mood so that didn't help. But when he failed he hugged me real tight and said he loved me. The thing is that he said it quietly and in a very earnest way, as if he was afraid of something. I don't know if Trev is unsure of me, unsure of how much longer he has me, afraid of the future.

Sally knows it is a dangerous game she is playing, that the costs could be high:

I don't want to destroy our marriage just because I am restless and I don't want to hurt Trev. I'm just not sure how much I can play around without causing a disaster for lots of people. Poor Trev, I am more compassionate to him now I think. I tolerate him more, knowing if I am patient there may be more out there for me to experience. Not just men, but life, doing things, seeing things. I just don't want to wait until it is all too late and I am old. I want him to think everything is OK, which it mostly is. Nice and safe and acceptable. It is just what is churning away inside me that is the problem. I know I will get caught out eventually if I keep this behaviour up but apart from hurting Trev, I am OK with whatever the future holds for me. I have spent all my life being so safe, but that is not living; that is just existing. 'I'm waiting ... for something to change my life, just like Didi and Gogo.' [She's been reading Beckett's *Waiting for Godot*.]

An affair can change your life. 'Those who are faithful know only the trivial side of love', said Oscar Wilde. Well, he would say that. But it is certainly true that illicit liaisons can offer amazing emotional intensity, heart-fluttering human drama—excitement beyond the wildest of whitewater rafting trips or knee-trembling bungee jumps. The attraction of the sexually illicit will always glitter, and good intentions fall by the wayside.

Many will say it is always best not to stray. Sexual betrayal deals a mighty blow to the trust that so many see as the bedrock of modern marriage. It is striking how many of my diarists mention the discovery of an affair as one of the reasons for the break-up of a previous partnership, and very few—nine of the ninety-eight diarists—mention an affair during their current relationship. Yet there's no doubt that a discreet dalliance helps some through dark times in a marriage, and makes a sexual drought more tolerable. Risky, yes. But only sometimes a disaster. Often this great adventure remains hidden—a cherished secret that causes no pain.

8

Two Pounds of Liver and a Cabbage

It's bedtime after a busy Saturday at a rural property near Bunbury in Western Australia. Ivan (aged seventy-four) is gently caressing his wife Suzie (aged sixty). He tells me they are both rather weary:

> As is normal, when we arrived in bed we embraced and kissed. To my surprise, I found myself getting aroused. We dawdled and played a little and something she said brought New York to my mind and I said, 'We've made love in New York a few times'. To which she replied, 'One in particular I remember. It was freezing cold and we stayed in bed in the morning and made love'. 'For quite a long time', I said.
>
> 'When you think of the time we've been together', I said, 'we used to make love up to four times a week and now we've tapered off but I'd say we've probably made love in excess of 3500 times. Some of it has been profoundly beautiful, some of it just beautiful, some of it just very enjoyable'. 'Yes', she said. And we both went to sleep.

Ivan and Suzie have been in this loving relationship for thirty-five years—many would envy them. The sex diarists include many people just like them, people who don't lose their spark for each other. We tend to forget they exist amid all the doom and gloom of couples struggling over their sex supply. 'I'm never going to get married. People are so horrible to one another', groaned my

20-year-old daughter after reading one of the early chapters of this book. I wanted to show her that there are couples in sexy, loving relationships that have lasted thirty, forty-plus years.

Some wrote to me wanting to be part of my research, not to help them sort out problems but because they are having such a good time that they wanted to tell the world about it. People like Ivan, who took heed forty years ago when a much older man, noting his commitment to business success, took him aside and warned him: 'Young man, don't neglect your wife's sexual needs'.

Ivan has never done that. He writes page after page of the lessons he's learnt from trying to keep the flame alive. 'Although I believe that men think about sex a lot, they don't give much thought to lovemaking', he tells me:

> In a civilised relationship, sex, or lovemaking, is a cocktail concocted from a need or a desire to copulate, mixed with elements of lust, affection, love, intimacy, humour and, especially, communication. Is there a more beautiful way of celebrating your being alive? The wonder of it. The excitement of it. The shared pleasure. Communicating that in an intimate and exhilarating way. But, it should be mutual. The light in the eye is essential. No light, don't go there.

He goes on:

> Remember the song 'Come on Baby, Light My Fire'? That can mean starting the mating dance hours before. If the signals are faint, I'll gently see if I can strengthen them … with a lingering kiss or a touch here and there. If there is no obvious inclination, then I won't push it. I'll back off. I look for tacit communication that she is in the market—or could be. The communication is in the eyes—and the way they look into mine. I can feel instantly if we're on the same wavelength. I can then be emboldened to make suggestions, like 'How's your skin at the moment? Does it need to be creamed?' We

both understand the code. We are both averse to being obvious and blunt. I prefer innuendo and teasing.

I don't like being knocked back so I avoid putting her in that position. This enables me to settle things down before they become too compelling. Years ago I would feel deprived and resentful—not any more.

He talks about the books he has read, including David Schnarch's *Passionate Marriage*.[1] He was delighted that Schnarch promotes making love with eyes open. 'I knew all about that', says Ivan. 'I thought I invented it.' He's spent years thinking about how to enhance and heighten his and Suzie's lovemaking experience:

> We installed a full wall of mirror in the bedroom. We made love lit by a small light, we kept our eyes open. We did each other. Within the one session, we would range from the intimacy of tenderness and caring to the intimacy of fucking each other. I adore it when she rides me and sits up, then leans back and then forward and sways so her breasts lightly brush my chest from side to side and again when she brings them up to tempt my lips.

The seduction takes place not just in the bedroom. Ivan loves buying her clothes: 'Somebody once said to me, "You're not entitled to take off a woman's clothes unless you've bought them". Well, I loved taking off her clothes and I loved buying the clothes that I would later remove—slowly'. When he travelled all over the world for business, he'd pop into boutiques and find something for Suzie—'She loves clothes and shoes. She loved what I bought her. I quickly learnt that my giving her clothes excited her. It excited both of us, especially when she gave them a trial run. We developed a cult of christening each article by making love with her wearing it'.

Suzie tells Ivan that he is her teacher. But his inspiration comes not from wanting to pass on experience, but from his desire to please her: 'It's because I love her and I want her to enjoy, to be taken over with an overwhelming pleasure—of which I am a part. Watching her relish the moment is an exquisite pleasure for me'.

Would that all women had such a lover. What shines through the diaries of loving couples such as Ivan and Suzie is such generosity of spirit, delight in each other's pleasure and gratitude for what they have achieved together. They count their blessings, all the more so when it hasn't been easy to achieve this long-lasting honeymoon.

Beverly has been married for twenty-six years to Ashley. They have had their bad times, particularly when they had young children and were running a business, and the stress was mile-high. 'I very much remember the creeping hand but I think what I hated about it was the fact it went straight between my legs or to my breasts rather than saying a few nice words to me', says Bev. But now everything is so much better.

Bev's husband works on construction projects for four weeks at a time, followed by a week off. She writes:

> After nearly nine months of this fly in fly out routine, we are more in love than ever and we probably communicate better than we ever did. My husband phones almost every night and we spend up to an hour talking … which is more intimate talking than we managed before. We make sure that our week together is planned to have lots of family outings and fun, with sex a priority on the agenda. We do our best to get as much in as possible and it gets 'juicier' all the time. If my period happens to fall on his R and R, that is OK … he is just happy to wrap his arms around me, but we still manage to sexually satisfy each other anyway. I think from it all we have learnt not to take each other for granted and how much we really do miss each other. It can only have positive effects too for our children to see how much we *have* to talk on the phone each night and how caring we are towards each other.

How do they do it? How do these people get through the tough times when so many of us flounder and end up distant and estranged from our partners? A few throwaway lines in the diary of 56-year-old Alice seemed to offer some clues. She has been married to Shane for thirty-four years—the Bathurst couple met when they were students—and they are among the most sexually active of all the couples who wrote for me. For the first ten years of their marriage they had sex at least once a day, often twice or three times. Now it averages out at about five or six times a week, although they still sometimes have multiple sessions in a day.

The first time Alice wrote to me, she mentioned times when she was angry with Shane:

> At times when we have been out of sync emotionally, I found it hard to be generous about sex but recognise that as soon as I let go of resentment and anger, I want to touch him and find sex a reassuring sign that we are back in tune. I hate being out of touch physically and emotionally with him, so I try to be constantly aware of words and actions which block us from that. This is about my maturity and letting go of ego rather than destructive submission or self-denial.

I wrote and asked her to tell me more. Her response was that their relationship is normally so good that she hates it when they clash and is always keen to try to recover their harmony:

> If I can remind myself that it is really *me* I don't like when I'm unloving, impatient and unkind, I start to calm down and pull off some of the prickles that are stuck on me at the time. I realise that I actually dislike myself more when I'm like that than I dislike Shane.
>
>   I think I decide that I want it to be good again, and the only way is to stop being cross. In this process I remind myself that Shane may not be ready at the same time as me to be friends again, but it is still worth getting started. Sometimes I find that

he actually isn't as cross as I was with him and my flying off
has been a puzzle to him. Self-righteous indignation can be
quite intimidating.

No matter what may have triggered the disharmony, I am
usually able to find something/s for which I need to apologise
to restore my own dignity and integrity, and for me that is a
good way to resume the conversation. Shane is definitely not
ungracious, but he doesn't 'say' sorry. He moves into 'being
sorry' as it were. I used to think that anger was OK and justified
if I was 'wronged'. Now I see that it is most destructive. I miss
out on all kinds of things when I slip out of gear in that way,
so I've got much better at checking out how things are going
relationally and if I've understood things properly. It has helped
to recognise that some of his reconciliation will be tactile rather
than verbal and to think about my tendency to use words to
control things to my advantage.

Now, isn't that what we should be teaching young people
in schools? Her words are a real lesson for life. As you might
imagine, reading this couple's diaries was a delight. They are so
happy enjoying each other.

Have a look at Alice's diary entry for 26 December. For days
they have had a house full of visitors, which means their daily sex
has been limited to early morning sessions—'quick and quiet'.
Finally, in the late afternoon, the guests leave and Shane suggests
'a rub and buzz session' (Alice usually needs a vibrator to climax—
that's the 'buzz'). Here's Alice's reaction to Shane's suggestion:

> Normally I like to finish the jobs that need doing before I feel
> like relaxing but it seemed like the perfect thing to be doing.
> So I was very ready to join in. I put on music and lit incense.
> I don't know who plugged the buzzer in for me, but it is a great
> encouragement for me when Shane does it because I know
> he wants me to really enjoy the sex and have an orgasm. It
> is an ongoing frustration for me that I can't orgasm without

other stimulation, although it is less of a priority now and I know probably the reality for many women. But that wasn't a thought at all this time, because my pleasuring was the main focus for both of us. It is such a turn on that he loves me to be pleasured.

At the start I was content with stroking and touching and probing, and then wanted to bump things along so reached for the buzzer. It seemed like we were both focused on me, which is delicious, but I also like to be touching his cock at the same time. I think there is a combination of not being too selfish and loving the feel of that gorgeous pole. After a while I was getting very self-absorbed and stopped touching Shane to work on my breasts and keep the buzzer in the right spot. Once I was on the downhill slope I couldn't think of anything else and so I went for it. I like to go for more orgasms after the main one, and he was great as usual about urging me on. Then I turned my attention back to him. I love extending my own pleasure with his, although I know there won't be any further orgasm for me.

In writing about the same session, Shane commented on how much he enjoyed giving Alice pleasure:

I really enjoy this activity, especially when Alice gets aroused and brings her wand into action. As she buzzes I do finger stimulation which seems to give her intense pleasure, leading to strong orgasm. I find this sexual activity immensely pleasurable even without any direct penis contact, although most times Alice will continue to rub my cock at the same time. I think this is a change from some years ago when I only got pleasure from direct stimulation and climax. Today my main thought was for Alice to get [an] orgasm and I would take my pleasure from that.

Here's Shane writing a few days later.

Tuesday, 1 January 2008—Shane's diary

I awoke with a very strong erection. My only thoughts were to couple up for some hard quick thrusting and climax. Very self-centred. We went for a long walk later that morning and when we got back our overnight New Year's guests had left and I asked Alice if she felt like some sex. She did. I was thinking of mutual massage and magic wand for her. I was on the bed first and when she came in we did some genital rubbing and rather than getting her wand out she started with exquisite mouth work, which I really love. It seems Alice doesn't need or choose to reach orgasm anywhere near as often as I do but I am happy to participate in whatever way she wants. Many times this means she controls the flow as I feel I should give her time to choose the wand according to her mood/arousal. After prolonged mouth work she took the on-top position and we had a really great fuck. I am constantly overwhelmed by her fantastic generous lovemaking.

Here she is, writing about the same day.

Tuesday, 1 January 2008—Alice's diary

HAPPY NEW YEAR! And it was. Once again we had visitors in the house and we mutually worked on very quiet sex in the morning, but in the afternoon after they had gone it was different. I asked Shane if he wanted to watch a DVD with me and was just finishing a couple of chores before settling down to do that. Then he asked if I wanted to do some sexing. I was OK about going with that but was on the verge of getting annoyed because he went straight to the bed, stripped off and just lay there waiting for me while I put some things away which I'd been working on. But I realised that I was choosing to carry on with what I was doing, not being forced to do it, and it was OK that he wasn't interested in what I was doing. I wasn't really that interested in it either. In the past I would have held a little (or a lot) of resentment about that and been grudging about my participation in the sex. Fortunately I've evolved a bit, and hope to keep learning so that I join in honestly and enjoy whenever we have sex.

When I came to the bed I asked him what he had in mind. He said nothing special, but I had this sense that he would like to be pampered, so I decided to do that. When he lies back and totally absorbs, he looks so gratified. This used to bug me—a rather self-absorbed, slightly smug and satisfied look. Now I'm happy that it is a sign of lust and absolute delight which is really a kind of trust and gratitude which I find appealing, and I love pandering to it. However, I imagine that if my needs and pleasure were not being attended to with devotion and generosity by him, I could get really resentful about this.

His absolute favourite pleasure is mouth work, so that's where I went and my cues from him were his groaning and his completely open body. He did respond at one stage by saying how much he loves what my lips do to him. After a while my mouth was feeling overworked, so I told him I was switching to my other 'lips' to continue the pleasure. By then I also wanted him to work on my breasts and buttocks so I didn't feel totally left out … I also prolonged the pleasure of the fucking for me by keeping the rhythm slow and steady for some time, until he wanted to release. Delicious!

There is much wisdom to be gained from this couple's daily negotiations over sex—her ability to seize the moment and make sex a priority, even when she had planned to do other things; his acceptance of the fact that she sometimes doesn't feel like becoming aroused or having an orgasm; the fact that they are both happy to tell each other when they are not in the mood but do always strive, where possible, to look after each other. And yes, sometimes he will 'just do it', rather than let her down:

No matter how non-aroused I might be, my feelings change quickly once Alice starts any foreplay. If she is showing interest in sex I always feel good about joining in. I don't have any resentment or negative feelings about just doing it—I feel very loved when she shows an obvious desire to share sex.

He also makes very obvious his delight in her pleasure, and is very willing to tell her how attractive she is to him. She revels in his body and her 'magic' power to make him stand to attention. How many men would envy Shane having this woman who is now so comfortable initiating sex and telling him what she wants. 'When we were younger I was often too embarrassed or uncertain to ask for specific help and just hoped he'd find my trigger spots by accident', she tells me, explaining that through years of careful observation by him and more assertiveness from her, they now enjoy much happier and freer communication about sex. This is a couple who really make love, day after day.

Wednesday, 14 November 2007—Shane's diary

Awakened this morning by kisses on my stomach and a hand caressing my genitals. As my erection grew, Alice smeared lubricant on me and herself, then rolled on top of me for intercourse. I lay mostly still while she did the rocking and rolling. This is very sensuous and I feel very indulged and loved when she takes such direct action.

Monday, 3 December 2007—Alice's diary

This morning I woke to Shane rubbing my back. I think I could lie for hours with someone rubbing my back without having sexual thoughts, but I feel selfish if I absorb it for too long, so I rolled over and indicated I was ready for more activity by opening up my bits and by joining in with my hands on him. It is aphrodisiacal to be wanted. Even if I am not aroused, I like to give and receive touches. Part of the pleasure is that he generously loves my body with words and sex and I love to love him.

Sustaining such a happy, active love-life is easier if you have a juicy tomato like Alice. Yet most women aren't like that. As I have shown, most women aren't so easy to please; many find that as time goes on, they become less interested in sex and are less likely to reach orgasm—the rewards aren't there for them. But that doesn't mean the end of an enjoyable, loving sexual life—provided couples are willing to adjust to these changes.

There were other diarists who showed that it is possible to achieve a harmonious sex life while catering to the ups and downs of the more typically fragile female libido. Take Sam (aged fifty-four) from Brisbane. He's the lucky man from Chapter 1 who wrote about his joy at being married to a loving woman who never says no to sex. Well, hardly ever. Rose certainly feels free to tell Sam when she's not in the mood, and he's alert to the times when she's too tired, stressed or uninterested. But she also enjoys catering to her husband's sexual needs, just as he makes strenuous efforts to support her in every way. So even when Rose is not in the mood for sex, she'll often respond happily to his advances:

> I do know that on many occasions I am a slow starter with little interest, but what happens mostly is the more we get into the act of sex, the more I enjoy it. I am as satisfied as I have ever been in my entire life. I love my husband and I know that having him sexually satisfied makes for a very loving atmosphere in the home.

Sam points out that his wife never initiates sex, though she 'always makes me feel welcome'. He struggles a little in trying to work out what she wants on any particular occasion:

> Often it is difficult for me to grasp whether Rose desires sexual release herself or is making sex a gift until matters are well advanced. Once I figure she is making sex a gift, I relax and enjoy. I have learnt then not to try to force the issue, not to attempt to stimulate her to orgasm.

Here he is writing about one such occasion.

Monday, 3 September 2007—Sam's diary

Rose went directly from work to her lead-lighting class tonight, so she didn't get home until late. It was close to 11 p.m. by the time we got to bed. By the time 11 p.m. did roll around, I was snoozing in post-coital bliss. This was one of those times that Rose made sex a gift. It was late and she needed to be up early to go to work, but nevertheless she made me welcome, despite the fact that both the need and the sexual release was all mine.

The next day he sent her a big bunch of flowers at her work. She writes:

The girls at work were fairly cynical about why he sent them until I showed them the card that came with them. The card read, 'Just Because', and then they all melted. Mind you, it brought a tear to my eye when I read it too. I am so lucky to have such a caring husband.

Sometimes when Rose plans to make sex a gift, her own reaction comes as a surprise.

Tuesday, 25 September 2007—Rose's diary

Sam came to bed with me. I had no indication that he had sex on his mind and I was not at all interested. I was tired and grumpy. I asked him to be gentler with his touching of me because I was just too tired to tolerate anything strong and vigorous. He gently persisted and I was very surprised that I reached orgasm. Once he got me there he entered me and we continued until he climaxed. We drifted off to sleep like a couple of well-fed puppies.

There are also times when *she* is dead keen.

Thursday, 16 August 2007—Rose's diary

On awakening Sam and I shared very loving cuddles and some touching without proceeding to intercourse, and we were both happy to leave it there but I knew that we would carry on with it that night. During the day I looked forward to it with pleasure and anticipation. After a relaxed evening we proceeded off to bed and basically took up where we left off in the morning. Because of the mental build-up during the day, our lovemaking was intense, giving and loving. I was satisfied to the point of euphoria and I felt that Sam was of the same feelings.

She knows how to handle him and understands he is keen for her to experience as much pleasure as she can. But sometimes all she wants is a quickie, so she makes sure that's what she gets:

Our next sexual encounter was yesterday. Sam was emailing me throughout the day with wicked suggestions of what he would like to do to me when I returned home from work, but I was having a particularly difficult day and soon lost patience/ interest. I thought to myself that if he was still in the same frame of mind when I got home, I would make sure our encounter would be fast and furious, thereby bringing us both to climax quickly.

He was in the same frame of mind and greeted me by leading me into the en suite, turning on the showers and only just gave me time to undress before dragging me under the shower. He did spend some time giving me a lovely neck and shoulder massage before moving on to anything sexual, but once started I made sure it was not going to go on for too long at all. Afterwards, he said that was not the plan and he had intended to make it to the bed and continue with our lovemaking. I had a little smile to myself because I got exactly what I intended. I love my husband very much but sometimes it needs to be my way as well.

Sam wrote to me feeling rather bewildered about what had happened, as he had intended to have a long lovemaking session.

It turned out that Rose hadn't expected to climax because she was tense after her tough day at work, but she still enjoyed it: 'It never matters to me if I don't because I am very aware that it takes a lot of just the right "stuff" to make me climax, but I am still capable of getting very excited'. She had been worried that if she said she just wanted a quickie, he would feel she just wanted to get it over with and would be disappointed. But it wasn't a big deal for this couple. He's happy to accept it when she offers sex as a gift, although he's still feeling his way, trying to work out exactly when this is happening. And she's gradually learning to trust him enough to be open about her desires.

This is one of the big issues that commonly brings other couples unstuck. While it's great to see how eager many men are to please their partners, that can put pressure on the women to feel they have to come up with the goods, even when they are not in the mood to respond. Many loving relationships work best when the quickie is part of the repertoire, which often will mean that the woman gives it as a gift, without expecting to climax. Many female diarists tell me this is fine by them. They are happy to just do it and don't mind if they don't get particularly aroused —provided there are regular opportunities for the prolonged lovemaking which does totally satisfy them. Many are happy to just give their men a hand job, or oral sex, instead of bonking. The real problem is their partners who, like former US president Clinton, seem to think real sex must include intercourse, and also don't understand that it is fine for many women to sometimes have a quick shag without climaxing.

Pauline (aged thirty-five) had been married for only five weeks when she first started writing for me, although the couple had been together for six years. She was still having trouble getting through to her husband, Daniel:

> I woke up when Daniel got out of bed. I had had a bad dream
> and needed a cuddle, so he got back into bed. I started kissing

him, and because we were so warm and cuddly I initiated
sex by asking if he had time for a quickie. He was happy but
surprised—we rarely have sex in the morning and it's nearly
never initiated by me. He wanted to have more than a quickie
but I told him we didn't have time. The truth was I wasn't in
the mood for a full-on thing. He was a bit sulky but was still
happy with what he got. Daniel likes full-on sex, which is great
once in a while but he would like this every time. When he is
horny he wants it all. I find it annoying that while we are having
sex, I feel that what we are doing is second best because he
always wants more. First thing in the morning with the child
sleeping in the next room is not, I feel, the time for bells and
whistles sex; it's time for quickie, snuggly sex.

As Alice and Shane have shown, it is possible to move past
these tensions by accepting that there will be times when the
lovemaking is directed just at him or just at her, and not always
expecting or demanding mutual pleasure. That's one of the keys
to getting it right.

But it is also very obvious that many women are missing out
on what they really prefer, which has more to do with touching,
caressing and holding than with what we think of as sex—namely
intercourse. As Barbara from Dubbo puts it:

> I do think though that there are lots of times when a woman—
> and this means me—only want to have a hug or a cuddle to get
> the feeling of closeness. But they always want to have SEX!
> I feel annoyed about this at times and I think why can't he just
> be happy to cuddle up in bed? I know it's not the way they
> work—their brains are in their dicks sometimes. They think
> straightaway that cuddling means it's on.

Then there's Mary from Perth. The forty-two year old remarried only four years ago, but already is finding that she has little
interest in sex. She knows just what she wants but her problem is
getting the message through to her husband:

What is my definition of foreplay and a good time? Tidy the kitchen bench and clear away the food scraps while I'm in the shower, greet me with the lights low in the bedroom, sheets turned down, him showered and smelling nice, a bottle of water or something nice beside the bed, and a long, long, long back scratch and neck massage. AND LEAVE MY BITS ALONE AND JUST LET ME GO OFF TO SLEEP—THAT'S IT!

But it doesn't make any sense to him—[if] there's no touching of the bits, for him it doesn't compute! It's like he gets stuck in an 'IF' 'THEN' loop with a glitch. So he just switches off and sticks to 'Plan A', which involves my nipples and the general clitoral area being massaged like he's kneading pizza dough.

I've often said that we treat others the way we want them to treat us. In the sexual sense I think it's very true. I know that the things Peter does to me are simply him doing what he'd rather I did to him; that is, focusing on stroking and playing with his bits. He couldn't really care less whether I touched his back or feet. If I spent a good hour playing with his erection he'd be the happiest man on earth. When he starts to mess around with my bits I feel like flogging him with a fly swat! I remarked to him recently that if he could figure out a way to give me a good back and neck scratch while doing me doggy fashion, we just might be able to work this thing out! I spend a lot of time giving him back scratches and rubs, all the while thinking 'do this to me'! Meanwhile he's turning into Houdini trying to leverage himself into a position where his bits fall into my hands so I can pay them some attention instead of his back—or giving me a good hint that the effort would be appreciated elsewhere.

Mary makes it very clear that she's over sex: 'In all honesty, Tina, I'm too old for this crap, I really am. I've had my kids, done my bit for mankind's continuity. I really would just like to put that part of my life behind me!!' But she'd be far more willing to offer her bits if her husband gave her more of what she really wants.

Yet, in the end, it is not just about sex. Years ago, when I was editing *Forum* magazine, I received a wonderful letter. A woman wrote to me saying she had read so many articles in magazines and none of them seemed to answer her problem:

> I have followed advice like '99 Proven Ways to Keep Your Man Happy' and 'How to Stay Young and Active Till You're 103 by Eating Sardines': have nearly crippled myself doing exercises to try to keep the flab down; practise positive thinking; clean my face every night and chew parsley to sweeten my breath. I have read so much about techniques, multiple orgasms and the importance of physical aspects of a relationship.
>
> I happily masturbate, fantasise, go knickerless and turn myself on at the biscuit counter at Woolworths, talk dirty, have armpit hair and turn out good lamb casserole. Come the weekend when I do not go out to work, I put on my make-up, do my hair and sometimes go braless in spite of the fact that at my age, my nipples shake hands with my navel.
>
> My house is the kind that Phyllis Diller jokes about: in other words, I do not put my dusting before screwing. I have never said, 'Not tonight, darling, I am too tired, have a headache/my ingrown toenails are playing up' etc., etc.
>
> Now accepting, as I do, the importance of sex—I know that when it is good everyone is relaxed and happy—I still wonder what happens to the other things attached to living together and bringing up children. Even when sex is good it still will not make him talk about money or do the garden or fix things around the house.
>
> It is kind of hard to lie in bed at night thinking, 'Shit, how am I going to make 1½ pounds of mince and three carrots last until Wednesday and John has not got clean socks for school tomorrow' and still feel turned on. Loverboy is oblivious to all this and then there is always the problem of money. Quite honestly, I would get turned on more quickly if instead of

playing with my nipples and caressing my bum [in] true *Forum* style, he would say, 'Don't worry, honey. I'll buy you 2 pounds of liver and a cabbage'.

It says it all, doesn't it? The other things matter. Irrespective of how good the sex might be, real life intrudes. The sex diaries make that very clear. And the couples who seem to be getting it right all talk about that total package—working on achieving real intimacy, no patronising, no ignoring of desires and whims, no assuming that 'I love you' excuses everything, treating each other as valued equals in all aspects of life.

9

Laundry Gets You Laid?

Mary has pulled the plug. She's put her husband, Peter, on starvation rations until he gets the message about housework. The 42-year-old Perth woman has been trying to get it through to him for four years, ever since they married; it was a second marriage for both of them. She's mad about the man. 'I really did win the jackpot when I met him', she says, explaining that her two children also love him dearly. And yet … there's a very big BUT.

'He just doesn't get the connection between housework and our sex life', says Mary, and then the stories pour out of her. Like the night she asked him to clear up the kitchen while she was working on her tax:

> He'd promised me he would do it in the 'ad breaks' on TV. At 11.30 p.m. I finished and went into the kitchen. He'd just moved all the dirty dishes to the bench around the sink, the dishwasher was still to be unpacked from doing the lunch stuff and there was gravy and crumbs all over the place. I said to him, 'I don't believe this—after all we've talked about this. WHEN are you going to get the message?'

He stormed off and, while Mary was unpacking the dishwasher and clearing up the kitchen, he went off to bed in their daughters' room. 'I've had a gutful', explains Mary.

I'm working a full 5-day week, 6 a.m. to 6.30 p.m. days. I come home, usually have to cook (because he cannot and will not cook, at least, not reliably). Occasionally he might put himself out but it's generally 'let's go to Subway', which I end up spewing about because I don't want the kids learning to rely on takeout and I spend a fortune each payday stocking up with fresh foods and meats. My weekends are guaranteed: all day Saturday cleaning the house itself, then Sundays attacking the ironing. Yes, he does 'do the washing'—which consists of putting the washing into our 10 kilogram washer/dryer, and putting the finished dried washing onto a pile on the lounge floor, where the dog promptly lies all over it. Now if he took the clothes out straightaway and hung them up or folded them, life would be sweet. BUT he piles them load on top of load on top of load—so by the time I get to them, I've got steam-dried, cardboard lumps covered in dog-hair and he wonders why I'm so bloody ungrateful and why that night I'll knock his block off when he wants 'it'.

Mary is absolutely bewildered as to why her man is allowing this issue to sabotage what she sees as an otherwise beautiful marriage. But Peter just doesn't get the point she's making and feels that it is incredibly unfair of her to use sex as a weapon. Mary explains:

He argues that even if I were a lady of leisure with a maid and housekeeper and no need to work, with a million dollars in the bank, I still wouldn't be interested in sex. I deny, deny and deny that but deep inside I have to admit there is a chance he is right.

There it is. That's the crux of the sex–housework issue. Yes, women are understandably resentful when they feel their partners aren't sharing their second shift. Why should they put out, 'just do it', if their partners aren't prepared to consider their needs and pull their own weight when it comes to the relentless burden of housework and childcare? The resentment these women feel is often a sure-fire passion killer. But even in the best of circumstances, even with the most considerate, helpful partners, the fact remains that many women still try to avoid sex.

Mary admits that housework isn't the whole story:

> Sex is simply no longer an activity in which its positives outweigh its negatives. It doesn't leave me breathless, it doesn't leave me feeling rested and sated. It just puts me in an awkward, embarrassing position and shows up all my bad bits: my fat belly, my flabby thighs, my boobs disappearing down my armpits.

She adds that her man still gets revved up just looking at her.

> Consequently I come to bed dressed in the most nunnish looking T-shirt night dresses and large white undies, and stick a Pillow Wall of China between us. I can play dead for as long as I like—he won't take the hint, he'll pester the living bloody daylights out of me until I give in. And then I feel like crap. I don't want it, but I'm forced to do it (just add 'sex' to my list of obligatory wifely and housekeeping chores—and how is THAT supposed to make me feel horny and sexy??) and because I really do love the man I don't want to hurt him but I just want it over with.

In her heart of hearts, Mary knows that even if Peter were to pull his weight around the house, he still wouldn't get what he wants. Yet that's not the message that men are receiving.

Look at what's happened to Dan from Brisbane. This 42-year-old man has been married for eighteen years and his sex life has long been in decline: 'It went from once a week, then once a fortnight … then once a month!' He decided to give up initiating sex and wait for his wife's advances. 'The first time I went four months without sex over Christmas and through my birthday. I knew something was not so hot then.'

His wife, Susan, won't talk about it without getting the huffs. 'Oh that's all you ever think about', she apparently says. 'Well, after a three-month drought ... yeah, funny, it is', is Dan's rueful response. 'We don't talk about it because it is never the right time. But it is eating away at me even if it's not affecting her. Now unfortunately we don't even do the hug thing because I've had enough of it', he adds sadly.

Dan says that he reads endless magazines and newspaper articles reporting that men who do housework get more action. He's tried that:

> We both work and I help out by picking up our little boy from childcare each day, cooking dinner every night, doing the washing, folding the laundry etc. I've been a Mister Mum for twelve months. I've tried all of those romantic ideas like hot baths and romantic dinners. None of this works. She can see it coming a mile away and now I do not put the effort in because I feel like it's thrown back in my face.

Then there's Fran. This 53-year-old Sydney woman is married to a saint, and she knows it: 'Julian runs the house, apart from cooking. He does all the washing but I won't let him do the ironing because he doesn't do a good enough job'. She knows he works very hard to try to make sure everything is running smoothly, in the hope she may want sex. 'Sometimes I think I'm such a bitch', she confesses with a laugh. The couple started off their 27-year marriage with a very active sex life, but then she lost interest: 'I see it as a chore and simply want him to get on with it. The thought of foreplay leaves me cold. I just want him to cut to the chase ...'

Julian (aged fifty-two) says most of his friends in long marriages also report that their wives aren't interested. But he's determined to keep trying and that means doing everything he can around the house to try to relieve her stress:

> I only make a sexual move at night if I think she has had a good day and all the indicators are on green. I think it is up to me to make things as appealing as possible and do everything I can to make sure there's nothing to put her off. But often this still turns up a blank.

He admits he feels pissed off and a failure when he can't get the sexual urge off his back. Yet occasionally he strikes gold: 'It's as if she's got these different personalities. If you get the sexy one, it's just great'.

They do talk about it, but as Julian points out, 'if I push the subject she gets very defensive and feels "invaded" and used. I cannot win so it's not really worth pursuing'. He adds that their marriage is not a 'void of lovelessness. There are plenty of hugs and kisses and the odd grope'. But Fran knows that he broods over the issue. 'I love him to bits. He really deserves a much nicer person than me', she says.

So what about the research that suggests doing the laundry gets men laid? There is some evidence of a connection. John Gottman, America's leading researcher on marriage, says that men who do more housework have more active sex lives.[1] Another researcher, Neil Chethik, has even quantified the amount of extra sex a man is likely to have if his partner feels he is doing enough around the house: one more session each month. His book, published under the catchy title *VoiceMale: What Husbands Really Think about Their Marriages, Their Wives, Sex, Housework, and Commitment*, grilled 300 American husbands about all of the above and found that the frequency of sex was higher when the wife felt that the division of housework was fair:

> Among wives who were satisfied with the division of house-work, two-thirds had sex with their husbands at least once a

week and only 11 per cent had sex less than once a month. When the wife was unsatisfied with the housework situation, the proportion having weekly sex dropped to 50 per cent and the proportion having sex less than once a month more than doubled to 24 per cent.[2]

What gobbledygook this is. There's a basic chicken and egg problem with all this sort of research. Isn't there a strong possibility that men who get more sex are more likely to have a smile on their faces and be willing to throw a mop around the kitchen floor or wipe down the benches? And it seems logical that when couples are close and connected, they are both more likely to share the housework and have more sex. Look at what happens when Dan starts to change the way in which he approaches his wife, starts to tell her how much she means to him.

'Had great sex last night', he wrote to me:

First time in over three weeks. It started off [as] a normal night, we were both tired and we went to bed about 10.30. I turned the lamp off and I let Susan start some arm's length cuddles. I responded with same and then we started light kissing. It was pitch black but I sensed her kisses were slightly different, more relaxed and 'lingering'. My hopes were up a little but I have been here before. The kissing continued along with some light touching. I told her I would like to make love and asked how she was feeling and how her back was. She said her back was sore so I took that as [meaning that] making love was off for the night. I asked if she would help me masturbate. It was dark and I found it difficult to gauge her response. I didn't push the idea and backed off. We kept kissing and touching and it escalated from there. It was a little while before I felt 'hang on she wants more'. I gave her lots of attention and next thing you know 'woo hoo'! I don't want to brag. Hang it, yes I do! We made love for over 1.5 hours. Started around 10.30, finished after midnight sometime. I counted Sue having somewhere between three definite and up to possibly eight orgasms.

So what was so different this time? Well, Dan had been working on trying to understand and connect emotionally with his wife, and here were signs that it was paying off. 'During love-making I was telling Sue how much I loved her and how good I felt making love to her, how it made me feel etc. Every time I did this the response was immediate and went up a notch', he says.

The interesting postscript to this was that the next day, Dan received a thank-you note in the kitchen, together with a request to hang the washing out. Dan's response was to tell her he just loves it when she uses the same note to leave sexy messages and detail house chores. Susan later confessed that she was giggling to herself as she wrote it.

So there it is—the couple move a little closer emotionally, and sometimes that leads to good sex and a big-heartedness that extends to sharing household chores. When you read the diaries of couples who are getting on well, this is what comes shining through. Men and women who really delight in being together are far less likely to quarrel about housework. They approach that issue with generosity and mutual caring, as they do sex.

Sam from Brisbane is one of the lucky ones. He boasts that he and his wife, Rose, are extraordinarily relaxed with each other:

> We care about each other, and each tries to meet the other's needs and desires, but this can hardly be classified as 'working on the relationship'. Rather, it is 'being in a relationship'. In large part, we take each other for granted. I know Rose is always going to be there for me sexually. She knows that when I am not on the road, that when she comes home dinner will almost certainly be underway and so on. Like most couples, we have certain routines about which we are largely unconscious. For instance, we discuss just about everything, but there are

areas where we both understand that Rose is likely to make the decisions and others where the decision will be largely left to me. We are comfortable with each other. This makes for a relaxed and happy relationship.

But it wasn't like that in Sam's first, 24-year marriage. In that relationship, sex loomed large as an issue, with his wife regularly complaining about his unreasonable demands. At one point, Sam decided to test out the notion that husbands who helped more around the house got more sex: 'I decided to try an experiment. For a couple of months I became the model husband. I cooked meals … I helped more with the housework. I took the kids off her hands to give her some more free time'.

The result? 'Our sex life got significantly worse', says Sam. 'If I cooked dinner, cleaned up, put the kids to bed and generally ensured she had no duties for the evening, the probability that we would have sex fell dangerously close to zero.' His wife would veg out in front of the TV and, in her sleepy state, be even less likely to respond to his advances.

Looking back, Sam now seems quite bitter about her reactions. 'Housework and tiredness are excuses, not reasons', he says emphatically, mentioning how he kept hoping things would get better:

> I kept looking forward to when the kids were bigger … when they sleep through … when they were all in school … when they are more independent … and so on and so forth, per tedium ad nauseam. All these milestones were passed, and our sex life failed to improve, despite the fact that my first wife did no paid work and had large slabs of leisure time during the day.

To men, such things as housework, tiredness and children can all seem like an endless stream of excuses.

Dan Savage is a widely syndicated US sex advice columnist. He recently commented that for years now, whenever he prints a letter from a man who complains about not getting enough, he's deluged by what he calls 'if only' letters from women:

> If only she didn't have to do all the housework, she would want to have sex. If only he would talk with her about her day, she would want to have sex. If only she weren't so exhausted from taking care of the kids, she would want to have sex. If only he didn't ask for sex, she would want to have sex.[3]

On the publication of Joan Sewell's book *I'd Rather Eat Chocolate: Learning to Love My Low Libido*, which argues that most women aren't interested in sex, Savage was delighted.[4] By proclaiming that low-libido women were normal, Sewell had done men a favour, Savage concluded:

> Well now, thanks to Sewell, straight guys everywhere know that it doesn't matter how much housework you do, or how sincerely interested you are in her day, or how much of the child care you take on: she still won't want to fuck you. So leave the dishes in the sink, grab a beer and go play a video game, guys. Your 'if only' nightmares are over.[5]

On one level he's right. Simply removing the sources of anger and resentment won't necessarily rekindle desire. But when these powerful emotions are still in play, men might as well forget about trying for sex. Hostility, irritation, resentment—all of these negative emotions erode the goodwill and generosity that is essential for women to feel receptive to sex. While they have us in their grip, nothing is going to work. Our problem as women is that we are just so good at chewing the bone, worrying over petty irritations and resentments. And our fragile libidos are easily distracted, crushed by the smallest niggle of annoyance and frustration, the tinniest flash of anger. 'We wrap up sex in all the garbage of the day', one woman once told me, and it is so true.

Listen to Barbara, a 58-year-old woman from Dubbo who has been married to James for thirty-nine years and has four grown-up children. She first contacted me after hearing me talk on the radio about couples fighting over their sex supply. She was driving along in her car with James when the couple suddenly found themselves listening to THEIR problem, the thorniest of the issues in their marriage, the one they never talked about. They sat in stony silence, listening to me prattling on, and when they got home she hurriedly emailed me to say how ghastly it had been to sit there, wondering what James was thinking.

Both Barbara and James had been married before. She was nineteen when her mechanic husband ran off with their next-door neighbour, leaving her with a 5-year-old boy and a 1-week-old baby girl. 'And I thought we had a great sex life', Barbara says ruefully.

Six months later she met James, and they clicked straightaway. Barbara says: 'We only had to walk past each other and brush an arm and it was like an electric shock. You'd look forward to going to bed and having a great time together. No hang-ups like there are now'.

Nearly forty years and two more children later, their sex life is just so much more complicated. 'I just don't want to do it', says Barbara:

Here I am, only fifty-eight years old, and I feel like my sex life is up the creek. If you have a lot of stress in your life, how in the hell can you even relax enough to want to do it? It takes so long for me to get in the mood, and the slightest movement, or thought, can turn me off in an instant.

Resentment is a big part of this couple's story. 'We have some problems at the moment with money', Barbara explains:

It's not that we are on the poor house doorstep but he just has this 'doggedness' about it. We have to be careful, he keeps saying. I'm not a spendaholic, and I agree with him, but I'm not going to go about denying myself a block of bloody cheese at the supermarket because 'we have to be careful'. You must think, what's this got to do with sex? It's got everything to do with sex, because it's these types of petty little niggling bloody things that make you resentful, and you think, 'Well, why do I bother to even be interested in sex?'

Sex just doesn't all depend on when you're in bed. It's the little things that are said and done during the day that count for me. If you're having a good day and there's plenty of talk and laughter, then I'm happier to agree to sex later on if we're up to it. Resentment is one of the biggest killers of marital bliss; it can creep up on you suddenly, like it did to me last weekend. Just little things start to annoy you and you think, 'Oh well, it's not so bad. He needs sex more than I do, so just let him get on with it and be done with. Doesn't really matter that your needs are being discounted, blah blah'. But then you think, 'It does matter! What's really going on here? It's just a one man band!'

Yes, women do add up the grievances; every petty irritation sets back their chance of relaxing enough for sex. But it's also that when they do end up in bed, pleasure can still be so elusive. 'He's so easily turned on. I'm not', says Barbara:

So you build up a brick wall that's impossible to climb over right from the very start. It takes me ages to get in the mood. I'm just so slow to be aroused, possibly because I can't relax enough. No doubt he's sick of me taking so long to be receptive. I would be, in his shoes. My mind goes all the time. When you are a mother it's very hard to turn yourself off from the lives of your children. I worry so much about what's going on with our kids, especially at night.

'Don't get me wrong, we still have a very good partnership', she says, explaining that they listen a lot to the radio and argue about current events: 'This is one of our foibles: we argue about each other's opinions, but there's a pretty high degree of respect for each other really'. And occasionally she still lusts after the man. She writes to me about their kitchen being painted and new slate being put on the floor: 'We're putting all the furniture back in. He's lying on the new floor trying to get the fridge back in its proper position. I'm standing watching and thinking, "Hmm, he looks pretty good down there. Wouldn't mind if we had a go on this new black slate floor!"'

And then she adds, 'But was it because he was getting in and doing something though? There's nothing a woman likes more than to see her husband DOING SOMETHING around the house, is there?'

That time she did nothing, just stood there and watched. But every once in a while, she does make her move—like the night she was up late, bidding on eBay for the Little Golden Books that she collects for her grandchildren. Her husband went to bed around 11 p.m. and over the next few hours she did well, scoring some much sought-after items online. She finally went to bed herself around 1 a.m., very happy and still wide awake: 'Of course it was no trouble waking him up for sex. He was only too willing, and very surprised, mumbling that he'd go and get some Little Golden Books every day if I repeated it'.

The ebb and flow of marital life endlessly batter and bruise what for many women is an elusive libido. But the male drive so often simply sails on, rising above it all. That's why men find it so hard to understand. Most women aren't using sex as part of a deliberate strategy to bribe men into behaving themselves. When a man lies on the kitchen floor manoeuvring a fridge into position, it may trigger that 'he's a good guy' feeling that encourages sexual generosity. But no, it usually won't get the juices flowing—that's a totally different story. And when a man simply increases his partner's workload by leaving crumpled clumps of clean sheets on the floor to be covered in dog hair, the ensuing irritation corrodes any of the goodwill that may just set the scene for foreplay.

'Just remember, when a low-desire woman feels burnt out, the first thing to go on her to-do list is sex', warns Michele Weiner Davis in her book *The Sex-starved Marriage*, one of the best self-help books available for people with mismatched desires. If a frazzled woman feels that she is being taken for granted, there is no way she's going to burn the midnight oil dreaming up ways to please her husband sexually, says Weiner Davis:

> If your wife has been one of those responsibility-laden people and her requests for help haven't inspired you to oblige, even if you think she is asking too much, you can't afford not to do it. Her resentment for feeling taken for granted will never go away on its own. You need to become more involved at home and show her you care about and appreciate her.[6]

That's the bottom line. Men who are determined to remain connected with their partners are more likely to notice when they are under stress, more willing to do something to relieve their load, and more likely to show appreciation for their efforts. And that means their partners will feel that they have a fair deal—no matter who does the most work around the house.

This is the complex picture we never hear about. Housework gets lousy press. Think about it. These days, whenever you read stories about who does what around the house, all you ever hear is the huge numbers of hours women put in and how little men do. And it's certainly true that there are women like Mary who are spitting chips over carrying so much of the load. But that's not the whole story.

For a start, when you look at paid and unpaid work, the total hours worked by both men and women in Australia are remark-ably similar. Most women work part-time; it is men who are putting in long hours of full-time work—which is one very good reason why research consistently finds that most women report that their deal over housework is fair, despite their putting in so many more hours on the home front. Professor Ken Dempsey, a La Trobe University sociologist who researched how women judge the fairness of their domestic workload for his book *Inequalities in Marriage*, had this to say:

> Women judge the fairness of their situations not just in terms of the time they or their husbands spend on childcare or housework. They take all sorts of other things into account such as the hours their husbands put into their work, their enjoyment in the nurturing role, whether they feel appreciated for what they do and, most important, their sense of emotional satisfaction in their marriages.[7]

At the end of my research, I received a final letter from Clive (aged forty-eight), who had been very frustrated when he first wrote to me six months earlier to complain that sex was a major issue in his marriage. The Sydney man had told me he'd been starting to wonder if he had a sex addiction: 'To be constantly refused, to not even try because you get fed up with being rejected. It builds up resentment, causes irritation. You start to think of nothing else. You want it more and more and you get less and less'.

The diaries helped him start to talk more honestly to his wife. He read the material I sent him, the couple gradually broke down some barriers, and sex became more frequent and more relaxed. Writing to tell me how much things had improved, Clive mentioned the housework issue:

> Cleaning the house I have found in the past has not gotten me any sex. I've helped—but mainly so I wouldn't get less than the meagre rations I used to get. As I'm now on steady and good quality rations, last weekend we had to do a spring (autumn?)

clean of the house. We recently had some good sex, and to me we were a couple—a loving couple together again.

I spent the weekend with her cleaning the house out and then washing the house down. Probably spent the best part of eight to ten hours over two days. It wasn't a problem. I was helping my lover and best mate and I wanted to be with her and I knew it made her happy.

What happened after that left him totally floored. Early on the Monday morning, the couple made love. Then, later that night, Clive was sitting at his computer:

I thought that she was getting ready for bed. Well, she turned up behind me wearing sexy red lingerie and invited me to bed—'Only if I wanted to'. Do I need oxygen? Again a … wonderful moment for the two of us.

Twice in a day—it must be over fifteen years since that happened. I felt like I'd just climbed Everest! I was so over the moon, and a big part was that she instigated the second one. We have come a long way since six months ago, when I felt like I was constantly begging for sex. She is far more aware of how important it is to me, and I'm aware of how she is feeling, and her moods. But I also give her a cuddle which she understands is a cuddle of love for her and not an overture for sex. Desperate and frustrated men do make many mistakes when it comes to sex in a relationship.

When Clive feels close to his wife, he wants to be with her, even if that means spending the weekend doing housework. And when they share these chores, it feeds the connection that will sometimes spark her lust. But there are no guarantees this will always work for him. The only sure thing is that, if he never shows he cares for her by sharing her load, then sex is likely to stay off the menu.

10

Get That Thing Away from Me!

The very idea of writing a sex diary was often greeted by mothers of young children with a wry laugh. 'Sex? What is that again? A no-sex diary is more like it', they would tell me. One young mother confessed that she has apparently mastered saying 'Get that thing away from me!' in her sleep.

The arrival of a first child often brings sexual strife in its wake. Statistics show that marital satisfaction plummets during the first two years of parenting, an occurrence which takes most parents by surprise. Harriet Lerner, author of *The Mother Dance*, explains: 'Nothing is more stressful than the addition or subtraction of family members. We understand the subtraction part, because loss is the most difficult adaptational task we deal with. But we underestimate the incredible stress of adding a new family member to the system'.[1]

The mothers who wrote diaries for me know all about that stress. Sheri (aged forty-one) is a busy Mount Isa mother with three young children. Sex rarely makes it onto her radar: 'I usually enjoy sex, once I get around to it. But for me sleep is a major commodity and takes priority over anything and everything else. My sleep debt is such that some days I just cannot keep my eyes open for anything'. Not even her birthday, as her diary from the day before the big event illustrates.

Saturday, 22 September 2007—Sheri's diary

It's my birthday tomorrow. My least favourite day of the year. I know Alec will be expecting some sort of celebratory sex and I'm not sure if I can deliver. Isabel has her dance concert this weekend—which is just a frenzy of hairdos, fluffy frocks and make-up. Ted's sports wind-up is today and I'm just stressed out. Sammy is feeling the effect of not being the centre of everyone's world and he's just being a whingey horrible child. Alec wants to have the family over to celebrate … and I know that will include my mum and that really gets me riled. I don't cope well with her in the same room. Who wants to have sex when you're feeling like this?

Sheri has a huge list of worries, but it seems that the very worst thing about her birthday is that her husband, Alec, will expect sex. And she's not wrong about that. On Sheri's birthday, Alec is still wishing and hoping that she might just come across.

Sunday, 23 September 2007—Alec's diary

Well the day has ended really well with family coming over for dinner and celebrating her birthday. Isabel's recital was a great success also and Sheri has a generally good glow about her. As always she looks as inviting as she can be as a result. I'm excited with the thought that maybe she'll want to celebrate her birthday. I can only wait and see if it eventuates. I'm not going to get my hopes up.

It doesn't happen. It rarely happens. 'Sex is not on my list of priorities and I can't even say that I miss it', says Sheri, explaining that by the time the kids are in bed, she's just so tired that she can't be bothered. But there are other issues:

I also find that spending all day with my children, all my needs for closeness, touch, cuddles etc. are fulfilled by them to the point where by the end of the day I don't want anyone to touch me, I just want to be left alone. I know Alec doesn't get that and he still craves affection and attention. He's like my fourth child. I need help and support from him, not another child who demands of me and drains more of my energy.

She says 'no' and he gets mad. And then his sulky behaviour leads to even more problems:

I also find that Alec's mood swings, determined by whether he's 'getting any' or not, are unbearable. He is almost impossible to live with when things aren't going his way. Door slamming, non-speaking, angry with the kids, sullen, sulky, inactive, over-eating—the list could go on and on. This just makes the prospect of sex just so much more unattractive, a vicious cycle, but the mood doesn't change until I give in and he gets his own way. I find his behaviour pathetic really. It just annoys me.

The more he pursues her, the more tension there is between them and the less likely she is to make the effort to get her head in the right place for sex. 'We lack the intimacy that we always had. I don't want to have sex with a stranger', says Alec.

Sheri's husband is now a stranger because motherhood has disconnected her from her eroticism, suggests Melbourne therapist Kaalii Cargill, who believes that women in this situation project their lost sexuality onto the male 'beastly sexuality', leaving the men with all the primitive sexual lust and the women with no sexual desire or passion. 'He is left carrying all the erotic energy of the relationship and continues to pursue. She continues to resist. Their relationship is now driven by her hostile anticipation of his pursuit', she suggests.[2]

Of course, men face their own issues when two become three. Men sometimes experience a loss of desire in the months following the birth of a child, reports Dr Bennett Gurian, a psychiatry professor at Harvard Medical School. Gurian found that while some men experience a sense of exhilaration from witnessing childbirth, others feel distress and guilt as their partners endure pain. Some are put off by seeing their partner's most intimate parts, their genitals, stretched and on display, and others end up feeling like an intruder. The strain and fatigue of caring for a newborn also often adds to a man's confusion and feelings of isolation, which can all impact on libido.[3]

Fatigue is a critical issue, suggests Sandra Pertot, a Newcastle sex therapist and author of *Perfectly Normal: Living and Loving with Low Libido*. Her PhD research investigated women's post-natal loss of libido and found that 50 per cent of new mothers reported becoming less interested in sex in the twelve months after childbirth, and 25 per cent reported a loss of enjoyment. As Pertot points out, the difference between these two figures shows that the main problem for many women is feeling like sex in the first place, even though many women with low libido are able to enjoy it once they get into it.[4]

It's not just fatigue, says Esther Perel, whose book *Mating in Captivity* reveals other complexities. Eros is redirected, she proposes, suggesting that women gain tremendous physical pleasure from their children. She's not talking about sexual gratification but, 'in a sense, a certain replacement has occurred. The sensuality that women experience with their children is, in some ways, much more in keeping with female sexuality in general'. Perel points out that female eroticism is diffuse; it's not localised in the genitals but distributed throughout the body, mind and senses: 'It is tactile and auditory, linked to smell, skin and contact; arousal is often more subjective than physical and desire arises on a lattice of emotion'.[5]

Perel describes the multitude of sensuous experiences that make up the physicality between mother and child: 'We caress their silky skin, we kiss, we cradle, we rock. We nibble their toes, we touch their faces, we lick their fingers … At the end of an exhausting day, a mother has nothing more to give but there may also be nothing more she needs'. A mother's intimate involvement with her children, all this fleshy connection, can so easily capture her erotic potency, to the detriment of her relationship's intimacy and sexuality.[6]

But there's also the fact that the whole experience of becoming a mother has such an immense impact on a woman's sense of self, her sense of who she is. 'Having a baby, even though you'd die for them, literally threw me for a sixer', writes 40-year-old Glenda from Adelaide, who has been married for ten years to Brian (aged forty-two). Her husband is extremely understanding—she describes him as a 'domestic god' and claims the man is living proof that there's no connection between the amount of housework a guy does and the amount of sex he gets. 'Mine does lots of housework and gets very little sex', she writes, spelling out how great Brian is around the house: 'He has no qualms helping with the kids. He's a great dad, doing housework, cooking, washing dishes etc.'. Yet she's gone from loving sex—'for the first year or so we probably had sex about twenty-eight times a week'—to just having sex to make her husband feel better. She knows exactly what went wrong, though. 'Children! Oh my goodness, what a passion killer', she says, adding, 'Yep, the mother thing has done me in'.

Glenda had difficult births, including 'a third-degree tear with my first child, that was a killer', followed by mild postnatal depression and a long period of feeling very anxious and physically very sore. She finally healed, but 'due to the anxiousness and tiredness it's never, ever been the same'. Her sex diary entries are few and far between, and always laden with guilt:

> Since my last report, we've done it once, just once. I had a prep mums dinner on Tuesday (30 October) and the topic of sex came up (of course!) and I was almost dared to do it that night when I got home. So I did! Probably one of the best ones we'd had for a long time but then I think, 'Well, that's good, that'll tide him over for a week or so, so I'm safe'. Groan.

Her domestic god deserves better, but sex has become just one more demand in her busy life. Even the thought of sex is enough to make Glenda shudder: 'I have this unwanted, annoying resentment which flows through my whole body, asking, "What about me? What do I get just for me??"'

British childbirth expert and anthropologist Sheila Kitzinger talks about the 'virtual annihilation of self' that can be associated with motherhood:

> When a woman turns into a mother she is treated suddenly as less, not more: she tends to be perceived by men, and by other women who are not themselves mothers, as having fewer skills, and reduced competency, intellectual capacity and commitment to all things that matter. Her identity has become that of 'a mother' and it is as if the rest of her—her working skills, her career goals and all her other interests—has vanished.[7]

Writing to me late one night, Sheri, the Mount Isa mother, mentions a conversation with a friend about saying 'no' to sex: 'We both came to the conclusion that it is because it becomes the only thing we can say no to'. Sheri goes on to talk about the fact that being at home with small children means that she has given up so much—'career, independence, choices—the list goes on'—but she quickly adds that 'it has been my choice and I am happy to have made my choices'. She is spending her time on things that have become important to her, such as making lunches, sorting out school socks, cooking and cleaning. But she finds that these things often seem 'so menial and less significant than what Alec has to bring to our lives'. A big issue for Sheri is that she feels there's often no recognition in her marriage that 'those small things have taken effort and care and have been done with love for my family and that they are not meaningless to me'.

So what's this got to do with sex? Well, this honest woman admits that in this situation, sex becomes power. 'It becomes something that can make a difference: it is that weapon [that] when used "well" makes him notice and makes him hurt', she writes, before adding, 'Uuugh! That is so nasty. The more I try to make sense of this, the more confusing it is. I'm going to bed!!' Sheri struggles to retain her sense of self as she drowns in the constant demands of her children and becomes angry at the man who fails to acknowledge her burden. Withholding sex is a means of flexing her muscles.

Part of the problem, suggests Esther Perel, is the willingness of women today to wallow in self-sacrifice for their children. She makes a strong case that our Western culture has taken the sensuous pleasure of caring for small children—a natural and universal experience—and inflated this bond to an astonishing degree. Childhood is sanctified so that one adult sacrifices herself entirely in order to foster the development of her offspring, becoming a one-person, round-the-clock child-rearing factory, Perel says, adding that mothers carry most of the burden.[8]

Perel also argues that there is something absurd about the extent to which couples' lives now so often revolve around their children. 'They never carve out the time and space they need to unwind and replenish themselves either as individuals or as a couple', she says, mentioning the absurdity of an open-door policy for the marital bed.[9]

In Sheri's case, there's not just an open-door policy, but a child permanently in the bed. Two-year-old Sammy sleeps with Sheri, while Alec sleeps in the children's bedroom. Sheri says:

All of our children have at some time slept with us but Alec's taken issue with it with this one, I guess, because of the lack of sex generally. Sammy is a bad sleeper and it just became easier for me to have him in the bed because I couldn't cope with getting out of bed to go to him hourly.

Alec is also a really bad snorer—so bad that he often woke the child—so he now sleeps permanently in the baby's room. Sheri acknowledges that this has its advantages: 'If I'm being honest it also gives me some respite from being constantly pursued for sex, so I really haven't rushed to do anything about it'.

Snoring and Sleep

Men, are you getting somewhat older, putting on a few extra kilos and partial to an alcoholic nightcap? If so, you may need to add snoring to all those reasons why your sex supply is shrinking. It was striking how many of my female diarists mentioned snoring as a factor in marital tension and decreased sexual interest. I had male snorers who'd been turfed out of the marital bed to end up sleeping on couches or in children's bedrooms, and cranky females who complained that their partners just don't take the problem seriously.

We often treat snoring as a joke, but for the long-suffering partners of snorers it's no joking matter. While people of all ages can snore, older men carrying extra weight are the ones most likely to produce the loud, thunderous sounds that can inspire murderous rage in even the most saintly partner. About 40 per cent of adult men snore, compared with 20 to 30 per cent of adult women. Alcohol, smoking, obesity and ageing all increase the odds of people becoming noisy sleepers. We're talking about a mighty big noise sometimes —some snorers clock in at 92 decibels, noise similar to that produced by low-flying jet aircraft. Partners can even sustain hearing damage from the really big boomers.

Snoring is *the* major reason why so many older women sleep badly, according to Dr Jenny Hislop, an Australian sociologist now working at Keele University in the UK, who's been studying older women's sleep patterns. She mentions British research showing that 63 per cent of women cite snoring as the prime culprit depriving them of sleep, with her own research showing that almost one third of women in their fifties report snoring-related sleep disruption three or more nights a week. Hislop found that women aged in their forties and fifties average six-and-a-half hours of sleep for every eight hours in bed. All those disturbed nights mean midlife marriages are producing some very grumpy, sleep-deprived women who are extremely unlikely to want to put out.[10]

Of course, women also snore, but Hislop's research shows they are often very embarrassed by the fact that they do so, and their partners are likely to be less tolerant of this night-time behaviour—female snorers are more likely to end up divorced.[11] Yet this is a problem which can be solved. There are now many successful ways of treating snoring, including the use of continuous positive airway pressure machines, a wide range of oral devices, and surgery on nasal, palatal, tongue or neck tissues, depending on which of them is contributing to the problem. Snoring is linked to hypertension, stroke and heart problems, as well as the risks of apnoea and dangerous over-tiredness—all very good and important reasons for snorers to seek help. But ending the misery of the grumpy, sleep-deprived spouse means she's just that much more likely to be in the mood for sex.

Speaking of sleep, it was also intriguing how many women commented that after orgasm, their partners quickly fall asleep while they end up totally wired. It's the extra oxytocin the men release at orgasm which leads them to feel very sleepy, suggests Daniel Amen in his book *Sex on the Brain*, adding that the same hormone is released in babies during breastfeeding, making them sleepy as well.[12]

But not everyone accepts this as the full explanation. There's been a lively discussion of the issue on various websites, with women pointing out that men are more likely to climax, leaving frustrated women to stay awake, left high and dry. Perhaps, but that's not always the story, according to some of my female diarists who complain that even after orgasm they are left wired, while he immediately nods off. The cheekiest suggestion came from males who proposed that men do all the work and expend more energy in sex —hence the exhaustion. Hmmm … my lively female diarists would quarrel with that one, but sadly the men might sometimes have a point.

It was striking how many parents ended up in similar situations. 'Sometimes I feel we've reached the hall sex stage', writes Sydney mother Lucy. She's referring to an old joke about couples having sex. When they are newly married, a couple starts off having home sex—all over the house, in every room. Then they progress to bedroom sex—only in the bedroom. They end up with hall sex—whenever they pass each other in the hall, they say, 'Fuck you'.

Lucy and Noel are both in their late thirties, married and with two children aged ten and twelve. A 'tree change' move to country Victoria has proven difficult, with Noel hating his new work situation and Lucy uprooted from her friends. Noel is keen for Lucy to return to the workforce to help out with the mortgage, but she can't imagine what she will do and how she will cope with work plus the demands of her family. So Noel works ever longer hours to try to dig them out of a financial hole while Lucy resents the fact that he never has time for the family or for her.

But sex, the difference in sexual desire, is the biggest battle-ground, where they play out many of their other tensions. Noel writes sadly:

> I desperately want to have sex and desperately want Lucy to initiate it. But alas, I am now becoming more stubborn and she won't give in to my needs so we become bitter and twisted with each other, only having sex when Lucy is in the mood or else feeling pity for me.

Lucy knows how dearly he wants it:

> As far as sex is concerned, I know he thinks about it all the time; he always has. I think about it too but am just not prepared to go to a place with someone who doesn't even hear me when I speak to him. But I do dream about him. Erotic dreams. It's this deep subconscious letting me know that I still love him even though things are so desperate. He's told me he can't touch me, not even a little bit, without wanting me. I feel that the minute I bridge that gap it's on and I can never keep up: the demand is just too great, and I feel so tired.

Looking back, Noel feels that the signs were there from the beginning:

> Building up to our wedding, Lucy started to make comments such as 'Most brides are too tired to have sex on their wedding

night'. It seemed like she was talking herself out of sex, or trying to convince me that it wasn't going to happen. Needless to say nothing happened. And yes it was a big disappointment for me. It's now what I remember the most about our wedding.

But in Lucy's view it all started with the children. 'I had no inkling motherhood could impact in such a dramatic way', she says, describing the intense tiredness and morning sickness, but, more significantly, the shock over the change in roles:

> As we finally emerged from this horror, life started to settle back down to an acceptable state. Sex returned again but now it was more like once or twice a week which was totally unacceptable to Noel. I did however 'service' him occasionally to keep him happy. This in itself created a new resentment. Not only did he still have a life, money, independence, but I was now relegated to chief cook and service agent. This is where I still am today. Our sex life is virtually non-existent because of the intense unhappiness I feel towards my treatment.

However, Lucy knows that Noel, too, is doing only what he thinks is right:

> Don't get me wrong—he's just as much a victim of this pattern that we've created for ourselves. I'm sure that in his mind he's doing what's necessary to make ends meet. Somewhere along the way it became evident that what each of us perceives as important is completely different. It's this lack of understanding that seems to be causing a major rift in our marriage. We still have sex occasionally and when we do it's almost desperate as though we are trying to recapture what we had.

Here's a woman who feels constantly torn between what's right for the family and what's right for herself. She resents what she sees as her husband's freedom:

Yes, his job is demanding—so demanding that his stress level is causing him illness. But on the whole he still comes and goes as he pleases, spends what he likes and makes decisions that he believes are OK, creating the feeling of him just being a visitor in his own home. It's these things that rot away in a marriage and the state of a marriage becomes measurable in the bedroom.

These are big issues for this couple, and they are not easy to resolve. But what stands out in reading their diaries is how much their world is focused on the children. Noel works desperately to provide for his family; Lucy has already been at home full-time for twelve years, caring for her children. They don't even use babysitters—'Noel doesn't trust anyone to mind the kids so we always go out as a family rather than as a couple'. Not only are there two curious older children ever-present in the house, but there are also dogs in the couple's bed. 'With two dogs in the bed, intimacy seems a little difficult', acknowledges Lucy.

So that huge gap between them in the bed is filled by their four-legged friends. That gap was never more apparent than the time Lucy wrote to say she had decided to try to fulfil Noel's long-expressed fantasy of waking up to her arousing him. She tried just that, but nothing happened. 'Unfortunately he was either just too dead asleep or not interested so I stopped when I got no response. I wondered whether he's just tired of the roundabout we seem to be riding or whether he really was too asleep', she wrote in her diary.

The next day she asked him about the previous night. 'He said he was awake but didn't want to respond as he wanted to give me some of my own medicine', Lucy explains, adding, 'Little did he know that it didn't bother me that much as I was doing it more to bridge the gap rather than for the sake of wanting sex'.

Interestingly, the diary process proved cathartic for this couple. At one point, Noel had what he called a 'meltdown'—in response to a comment I made about how sad he seemed—and the couple talked and talked. 'You're here in third person', Lucy tells me. 'I don't know why this seems to make talking easier but it's like we use the material we've provided so far as a basis to talk more openly. His willingness to talk now has opened a new doorway and it feels as though we've turned a corner.'

Lucy and Noel are still experiencing ups and downs but there have been moments of closeness, as she describes:

> Last night he made an effort to be more considerate of me by coming and saying goodnight with a hug and kiss. He also said, 'I'll be awake if you want me'. So I made an effort too and climbed into bed to have sex. It was good, but I was still very aware of all that's been going on and couldn't quite let it all go. His touch was far more tender, which is what I'd said I wanted, and I felt that it was more rounded, giving and receiving on an emotional level as well as physical, as opposed to the primal sexual gratification that we'd been creating in the past. He held me all night like he'd really missed me, and at that point I wondered if I'd been so callous as to not recognise his need to be held himself.

The really surprising thing is that while many young parents end up bogged down in sexual issues, others just sail through. Shirley and Luke are from Mildura; she is forty-seven and he is fifty. She mentions a time when they were young, when they ended up having sex while her husband held their crying baby. 'We finished in the doggie position so he could rock her and still get on with coming', she writes. They now regularly have sex in the bathroom on weekends when their teenage children are at home. It's often in the shower, 'usually in the standing position, taking her from behind,' explains Luke. Shirley writes in her diary about having sex on a Saturday afternoon: 'I was in the shower thinking I would like sex when Luke came and said he would join me'. There was a slight problem—their daughter kept talking to them through the door. Shirley acknowledges that 'sort of threw the moment as well. We just got it over with'. How's that for not letting the presence of children cramp your style?

Perhaps it is the women with stronger sexual drives who are less affected by the experience of motherhood. Claire (aged thirty-two) fell pregnant the first time she had sex. She married at twenty and since then has had three children. Although she felt lethargic during her pregnancies, motherhood has done nothing to dampen her libido: 'I have always had a fairly high sex drive and love of sex'. Even with young children, the frequency with which Claire had sex with her husband, Geoff, quickly settled into a pattern of three or four times a week, which suited him but left her feeling she had missed out. Now, twelve years later, they have scaled it back to three or four times a month. 'I am unhappy with both the frequency and the quality of the sex', she says.

For her, children have never been a big issue:

We snatch moments during the day when the kids are occupied—in front of the telly, playing outside—and we have a quickie somewhere, no foreplay, usually standing up in the bathroom, so I don't usually get there. I don't mind. It's still fun and if it weren't for these sessions, we'd have virtually no sex life at all.

Claire is very frustrated that her husband so rarely initiates sex, and she makes do with her vibrator. Here's a typical diary entry:

Last night I had to do some work and that took until about 10 p.m. Geoff was asleep on the couch so I masturbated before I went to sleep. I got there five or six times, and had a very nice sleep. I felt a fleeting sense of disappointment that Geoff wasn't awake but then I dismissed it, saying, 'Typical'. At least my vibe never says no.

At the other extreme there are women like Monica from Sydney, whose children heralded the slow death of her sex life. Monica (aged fifty-seven) has had no sex for the past three years—in fact, not only no sex, but no cuddles, hugs or physical closeness at all. When you talk to this funny, warm, friendly woman, it is obvious how guilty she feels about it, particularly since her husband, Greg, moved out of their bedroom and started sleeping in another room:

> The more I write the more I dislike myself, but withholding sex was never an intentional act. It just happened after two awful sessions of bump and grind which led to the long period of uncertainty and me thinking, 'Oh God I hope he doesn't want sex tonight?' etc. until he took action by moving into the spare room where he has slept ever since.

She knows it is wrong: 'It's such a pokey little room. He is a lovely, kind man. He doesn't deserve to be unhappy'. It was having children that caused her to go off sex, she says:

> The impact of children was HUGE! Once I had my two babies I felt that my body belonged to them and I have since found it repulsive that a grown man still needs to nuzzle like a baby, and the whole performance and mess is repulsive to me. It's as if I changed from tart to mother and the roles have remained separate for me.

This is a woman who reports having a wild time back in the 1960s: 'I was quite a demanding partner when I look back!!! So as soon as the penis was up I was ready'.

Twelve years ago Greg wrote her a long letter, demanding intimacy. She fobbed him off and sex has never been mentioned since. Monica is perfectly happy without sex:

> I think I feel contempt towards men for being so needy. I carry guilt every day but I have no sexual feelings towards him

whatsoever. To be honest I feel liberated without sexual activity in my life. It is as if I have risen above it. Does that make sense? … Something like moving onto a higher plane.

The couple has had counselling but neither was keen to discuss private sexual matters. There are complex background issues here. Both come from families where there was absolutely no physical affection, and Monica suspects something more: 'My father may have treated me inappropriately when I was little. I hesitate to use the word "abuse" but I think I was a troubled child. I have vague disconcerting memories but he and my mother are both dead and I don't feel able to "go there"'.

As is often the case, children are really only part of the story. But what is fascinating is the very clear shift in power in Monica's marriage. She is surprised to find herself with the upper hand: 'He used to be the powerful one but is no longer. I have all the power'. She kept thinking he would find the situation intolerable and leave her when the children grew up, but it never happened. He buys her expensive presents; he plans their future together.

She now says she finds it impossible to feel any desire for him: 'I have emasculated him by turning off the sex supply'. The result is that she sees him as lonely and pathetic, 'although I suppose he is in reality strong for not giving in to his desires and for hanging in there. But what is he hanging in for?' She ponders the idea that perhaps he feels insecure now that she is calling the shots, now that she has gone back to work and is doing her own thing. 'Perhaps he'll comply with anything rather than be alone', she adds sadly.

Men know exactly why they are hanging in there, wishing and hoping for change. It's because the alternatives are frightening. With divorce all around us, men understand that breaking up a family means they lose out, financially and emotionally, and, most importantly, they risk losing contact with their precious children.

My male diarists wrote so passionately about how much their children meant to them, the pleasure they had brought to their lives. Even as they bemoaned the loss of sexual intimacy that came with the patter of little feet, fatherhood brought its own, huge rewards.

11

Blind Man in the Dark Trying to Find a Black Cat

Ten years ago, Canberra couple David and Margaret, both in their sixties, were seated in a urologist's office, discussing forthcoming surgery for David's prostate cancer. The urologist came out with a surprise question. 'Do you like being poked?' he asked Marg.

It was a very good question, even if it could have been phrased a little more delicately. The urologist was trying to find out how Marg would feel if David was unable to have erections after the operation.

Well, it turned out that Marg was delighted at the prospect. 'I realised I would be quite relieved if there was not this third body in the bed to rear up with its hard demands just when I was enjoying a cosy cuddle', she said, explaining that intercourse had never been her favourite part of sex and she couldn't climax that way.

That was a major turning point in the relationship. David was a little miffed at the time—'It did make me wonder why I had been trying so hard all those years [to make intercourse pleasurable for Marg]'. He ultimately decided to forgo medication to give himself erections, but is perfectly happy with what he calls 'outercourse': caressing, touching, oral sex. And he still has orgasms—'even stronger than before!' he says, although he has them without an erection or ejaculation.

The couple say that as a result of plenty of talk and making adjustments, they have a new closeness and their sex life has never been so pleasurable. Marg says:

> Our sex life has got better and better. That's because I feel better understood and accepted for who I am while David is getting more of what he wants—physical contact with me—which I am enjoying more than ever before. The more I enjoy it, the more responsive and initiating I am, the more confident he is that I love him and the more he can enjoy the sex we are having without dwelling on the sex he is not having.

'I never thought sex in our sixties would be so enjoyable', adds David.

But sex for this couple has not always been smooth sailing. Initially, their sex life fell far short of David's expectations as he struggled with Marg's lower drive. 'He didn't want to accept that my sexual appetites were smaller and very different from his. Sex often just bored me', says Marg, describing years of tension, sulking and anger. Intercourse was always an issue: 'I used to have to work pretty hard to get any pleasure from David being in me. The right parts of my anatomy weren't getting the stimulation. God knows, he tried!' And David could never understand why it was so difficult for Marg to tell him what she wanted.

Now, finally, they have learnt to understand each other, with the work they have put into their relationship paying off in their physical relations as well. Yet their diaries show that the process of negotiation over lovemaking never ends. David isn't hard to read. 'He is very good at saying what he wants', says Marg, listing his preferences. But she says that she is never sure what will work for her at any particular time:

> I hardly ever know whether I will want to go further than stroking and a cuddle, or what is likely to turn me on until I'm

well on the way—or ready for sleep. Sometimes the stroking, a memory, a position or a fantasy will get me purring and looking for more. At other times, the very same things have no effect or irritate me. That makes it very hard for him.

Here's a typical diary entry from David:

Six a.m. we half woke. I didn't have a strong sexual expectation because yesterday was good and I still don't push my luck! We mutually cuddled as usual, then M moved her breasts for me to touch, kiss and suck. I enjoyed this for several minutes to the point where I sensed that she had had enough. At this point I asked if she just wanted to cuddle and she said 'yes', so most of my touching was sensual. After maybe twenty minutes, by moving her hips and legs, she indicated that she would like the touching to be more sexual. So I slowly began more touching of pubic hair, thighs, back, bottom, clitoris. Gradually she began touching my nipples (I have very sexually sensitive nipples) and we moved to mutual stimulation/masturbation for maybe thirty minutes, each having an orgasm.

He explains that he is now much better at reading her cues and is prepared to go with the flow:

Our sexual negotiation as you can see isn't just a 'Yes' or 'No'. I used to get frustrated by what felt like several start/stops. For decades I felt a mixture of confusion, rejection, frustration, anger and would have turned off, turning away from M in bed and sulking. When we have talked about this over the past fifteen years, it is clearer to me that she likes spontaneity, she is happy to be 'seduced' at times, and she says she never knows what she is going to want so how can she tell me beforehand. Fortunately for me, I now respond from moment to moment— I don't get frustrated. All of this is in the current context of knowing that, on balance, I will get enough sexual activity to be happy and satisfied. And of course I love being with her as an all-round person—she is an absolute pleasure to live with!

So this loving couple, after forty-three years of pleasuring each other, are still learning. Lovemaking simply isn't easy to get right. It isn't easy to learn another's body, to pick up clues on what pleases at any particular moment, to cater to another's changing sexual whims. We often don't feel safe enough to voice what feels good and what irritates, to share hidden desires. It is no wonder that so many couples flounder.

And there's a particular problem when it comes to women— we just aren't easy to please. Getting it just right with a woman can be a mighty tricky business. Twenty-five years ago, British agony aunt Irma Kurtz wrote:

> Naturally, women think their own loving, languorous way of sex is better, and so it is … for them. Recently they have been trying to bully and shame men into thinking it would be better for them too, though the truth is it would be less demanding, enslaving, perplexing and strenuous for a healthy male to screw a thousand women in his lifetime than to try to please one, and the potential for failure would be less.[1]

In Lionel Shriver's novel *The Post-birthday World*, Irina's partner, Lawrence, is surprisingly good at pleasing her, despite the impossibility of the whole project:

> His earnest manipulations were never quite right of course— never quite, exactly right. But to be fair, there was something inscrutable about that recessive twist of flesh, if only because the clitoris was built on an exasperatingly miniature scale. For a man to get a woman to come with the tip of his finger required the same specialised skill of those astonishing vendors in downtown Las Vegas who could write your name on a grain of rice.[2]

Shriver's heroine thanks her lucky stars that she was not a man faced with this bafflingly twitchy organ whose important bit measures not a quarter of an inch across, and chances are the woman herself couldn't tell you how it worked:

Because 1 millimetre to the left or right equated geographically to the distance from Zimbabwe to the North Pole. Little wonder that many a lover from her youth who had imagined himself nearing the gush of Victoria Falls had, through no fault of his own, been paddling instead the chill Arctic of her glacial indifference.[3]

That Arctic chill is something that many men know all too well. 'I have been trying for thirty years to stroke her clitoris the way she likes it but she says I am too rough or not doing it right. She always takes care of her clitoris and I stroke her elsewhere', writes Arthur (aged sixty-three) from Perth.

'Trying to find the right place on a woman's clitoris is like the blind man in the dark trying to find a black cat that isn't there' is another man's weary response.

Women know this. Every woman who has struggled to reach orgasm will have tormented herself with the idea that her lover is finding the process tedious. 'I start to worry about taking too long and him getting bored or even going to sleep', Phoebe tells me, adding that her husband, Larry, has actually dozed off in the past, which left her feeling sad and embarrassed. When women worry about whether his jaw is aching, or wonder what's going on in his head—'Isn't she finished yet?'—it makes them even more anxious and the elusive orgasm just slips away.

British comic Jenny Lecoat captures the problem this way: 'He, labouring away, pauses to ask, "Are you nearly there?" "It's hard to say", says she. He plunges on. "If you imagine it as a journey from here to China, where would you be?" She considers. "The kitchen."'[4]

In her book *I'd Rather Eat Chocolate: Learning to Love My Low Libido*, Joan Sewell acknowledges how impossible it is for men to keep women in the Zen-like, anxiety-free state needed for arousal and orgasm. Getting a woman aroused and responsive during sex is 'like building a fire in the damp woods on a windy day', she says, admitting that with her it's a lost cause. 'My libido is not very strong. It's as fickle as hell. It's apathetic and it's not easily aroused or easily sustained', she writes, adding that she does have orgasms, occasionally, but they feel like she's 'planted the flag on Everest … as far as the effort to get there, a lot of times it is not worth it'. Sewell concludes that this is all pretty normal for women.[5]

Yet masturbation is different. As Sewell coyly admits, she has 'bowed her own violin and can get her own strings to sing like Pavarotti'. For many women, an orgasm is not so elusive when they stimulate themselves. 'We know how to hit the right spots every time. We know how long to spend in this or that area. The right amount of pressure. The right type of motion', says Sewell.[6] But when she's with her partner, it isn't so easy: 'Even if I could allow myself to become sexually aroused in a relaxed non-judgemental way, that other adult squirming around breaks my concentration. My libido can't take distractions, or it just walks off leaving my body as passionless as a dead trout'.[7]

Sewell nails the problem pretty well. For many women it is not just a question of whether the man makes love to her in the right way; his very presence distracts her, worries her, makes her anxious and slows down arousal. 'I feel I am catering a party', Sewell explains. 'I'm not a doormat; I'm a welcome mat. In hostess mode I can't enjoy the party: I'm too worried about how the guests are doing'.[8]

That's where many of the sex manuals get it wrong. 'If a man could understand and become skilled in the ways that stimulate his partner to orgasm—then logically she would climax nearly every time they had sex together', write Marcia and Lisa Douglass in their book *Are We Having Fun Yet? The Intelligent Woman's Guide to Sex*. The Douglass sisters are obsessed about the orgasm gap, the infuriating fact that men get off in sex so much more often than women do. They are convinced that the problem is too much bonking: 'The low rate of orgasm for women is correlated with the high rate of intercourse-oriented sex. Intercourse simply does not give enough direct stimulation to the clitoris for orgasm to occur for most women'.[9]

Well, yes and no. It is certainly true that, all too often, sex consists of just the main course and not enough hors d'oeuvres. The data from the *Sex in Australia* survey revealed that 95 per cent of sexual encounters include intercourse, with men almost always reaching orgasm but women far more likely to miss out. The researchers, led by Juliet Richters from the University of New South Wales, conclude that it is the heavy concentration on intercourse as 'the central, almost compulsory sexual practice' which makes the difference. Women are most likely to climax when the menu offers variety, including cunnilingus, but too often women are stuck with the basic meat and potatoes, which doesn't do much for them.[10]

Yet, as Sewell shows, the reason that a woman may have trouble climaxing may have more to do with what's between her ears than whatever intricate manoeuvres a man may be performing on her clitoris. It's nonsense to suggest that the truly attentive lover can get it right every time. But it is true, as the diaries reveal, that sometimes women aren't receiving the attention they need.

Take Shirley and Luke from Mildura. After twenty-seven years of marriage, neither is particularly happy with their sex life. 'I have a really crap sex life', Luke (aged fifty) tells me:

> Wifey doesn't climax for me. I've tried for twenty-seven years and now sex with her … always ends with me feeling bad. I can grind away there for forty minutes or so and when I can't last any longer and climax, she gets cranky. I think I still love her but the thought of sex with her is not always a turn on. I've

had a fling with a woman who climaxed like nothing I've ever seen before. Completely orgasmic … Now I shy away from engagement [with Shirley] unless I'm really toey and need to feel a woman and not my own hand.

But Shirley (aged forty-seven) tells it rather differently:

He complains as he thinks he needs a marathon to get me off. I keep telling him he doesn't have to. It's all in the foreplay. He withdraws to stop himself coming and then my build-up is lost. How can I get excited about that? It's like once he gets going just get it over with. I may have a bit of pleasure in there somewhere and I try to tell myself it's good but it's just going through the motions. That's not what I want. I have given up on telling him what I want as he goes back into the just do it his way or no way. Not the good listener.

Ships that pass in the night. This type of diary makes for sad reading, as it reveals how couples can fail to connect and each partner is left feeling that they are missing out. I had wondered whether the couples who experience bad sex, sex which leaves them feeling deprived and disappointed, were less likely to retain their drive, while good sex might encourage repeat performances. I think that is basically true. But there were also women with no drive who said they had wonderful, attentive lovers, while other women lined up again and again for indifferent sex.

What is obvious is that the 'think clitoris!' message has well and truly sunk in. It was striking how many couples simply accepted that climaxing during intercourse wasn't going to happen and found their own ways around it—by adding a helping hand or bringing the woman to orgasm first and only then starting to bonk, or avoiding intercourse altogether and enjoying other treats.

And then there were the vibrators. It was amazing to discover that these helpful gadgets are now an accepted part of the sexual repertoire for so many couples. Thirty-five years ago I wrote my master's thesis on the use of vibrators and masturbation to help women who had never climaxed, which created quite a stir at the time. So it was very nice to now find that so many diarists felt comfortable employing this technology to make sex a little easier.

Here's Shane (aged fifty-eight) from Bathurst, who has been married to Alice (aged fifty-six) for thirty-four years:

> Our sex life started to blossom when we came by Alex Comfort's book *The Joy of Sex*.[11] This opened up a whole new world of sexual activity and more significantly much more communication. Mutual and shared masturbation and use of vibrators were great experiences, especially as Alice was able to get great orgasms with masturbation and/or external electric massagers. We have worn out a couple of these and currently have a Hitachi magic wand which seems to work best of all. Straight intercourse doesn't do it but the wand with or without concurrent intercourse works well.

But despite all this talk about clitoral stimulation, there are still plenty of women who respond well to a good old-fashioned bonk, as my diarists clearly show. When I asked women how they climaxed, many reported that the vagina did it for them.

Claire (aged thirty-two) says:

> I rarely get there without having sex [intercourse]. I could count on one hand the number of times a man has made me come with his fingers alone. I can get there with oral sex but I find that when these activities are good, they just warm me up, to get me ready for the main event—fucking. When foreplay is bad, I feel like asking to skip it altogether.

Gay (aged thirty-six) reports:

> Bart is the first man that has led me to full orgasm through penetrative sex. I love sex and I have had lots and lots of it

in my life with many, many men; however, I rarely reached orgasm. Usually just when I am getting there the man moves or comes. Bart is able to keep going. He can maintain an erection for one hour with no problem. He can orgasm several times and continue to have sex. He has a large penis and it must just get to the right places because I am very satisfied after having sex with him. He will always keep going until I have orgasmed at least once if not twice. No matter how much I move or push or squirm, he just holds on.

And here's Jill (aged twenty):

With Simon, I reach it about 90 per cent of the time. I think it has something to do with his shape—it's a little more curved than the others were. And, I think I'm more relaxed, I take what I want, not wait for them to give it. How? Rarely through oral, most often with me on top, sometimes with him on top. Never in another position.

The stories these women tell are being drowned out by the clitoral clamour. Everyone is working so hard to reassure women that it is fine not to come during bonking, that the women who do come barely get a mention.

'The tongue is mightier than the sword', argues Ian Kerner in his book *She Comes First*, which promotes oral sex as women's favourite sexual activity.[12] That's fair enough—oral sex works well. There's nothing like a wet tongue and soft lips to provide just the right touch for the delicate clitoral glans. But Kerner, like most writers of modern sex manuals, makes the mistake of putting his faith in research by Alfred Kinsey which declared that the clitoris was the route of all female pleasure and the vagina a sexual dead end.[13]

That's total nonsense. Kinsey, a famous US sex researcher, reached these conclusions back in 1953 using a team of gynaecologists who compared the sensitivity of the clitoris and the vagina using a cotton bud! It's hardly surprising that fireworks can result from cotton buds tickling the sensitive clitoral glans. However, it was recently discovered that the vagina is a very different beast. In 2003, British scientist Catherine Blackledge, in her book *The Story of V*, described research showing the vaginal walls to be richly innervated and capable of detecting vibration, touch and pressure changes. Here, the trigger for orgasm is vibration and deep (rather than surface) pressure, which occurs during the rhythmic rock and roll of coupling.[14]

It took a good forty to fifty years for us to recover from the era which followed the Kinsey pronouncements, which Germaine Greer called 'veritable clitoromania'.[15] It didn't help that Shere Hite declared clitoral orgasm the 'real orgasm'. Finding that only 30 per cent of women regularly climaxed during intercourse, she claimed they had to be deluding themselves. 'The pattern of sexual relations predominant in our culture exploits and oppresses women', she wrote, claiming it was a myth that penile thrusting in the vagina could cause orgasm.[16]

By the end of the twentieth century, for some feminists, intercourse had come to symbolise male brutality. Anti-porn crusader Andrea Dworkin—'I am a feminist, not the fun kind'—really put her boot in. Her book *Intercourse* describes the sex act as 'a means of physiologically making a woman inferior; communicating to her cell by cell her own inferior status, impressing it on her, burning it into her by shoving it into her, over and over, pushing and thrusting until she gives up and gives in'.[17] Whew! Certainly not the fun kind.

While Dworkin was ranting against the bonk, sex researchers were making some startling discoveries about what actually goes on during it, using couples who were brave enough to have sex inside MRI machines. When this work started, Dutch scientists had to use very slim couples because the MRI tunnels were a very tight squeeze.[18] But later they switched to machines with open magnets, allowing for more space and more vigorous action. Dutch and French researchers subsequently produced magnetic imaging showing the fit of the genitals during all this activity, and have come up with a few surprises. In the classic missionary position, the penis turns out to be bent like a boomerang, bringing it nicely into contact with the front wall of the vagina—the home of the famous G spot. And there's evidence that the clitoris is being stimulated both inside and out—through the vaginal wall, as well as via pressure from the man's pubic bone.

Around the time this research was being conducted, Melbourne urologist Helen O'Connell published her influential work on clitoral anatomy, showing that the clitoris is not just a tiny button near the vaginal opening but a large, expanding, highly sensitive structure which extends up to 13 centimetres and curves around the urethra and vagina. The entire clitoris contains spongy erectile tissue, similar to that in the clitoral 'glans'—that's the bit you can actually see, the 'magic button' visible just above the opening of the urethra (or urine pipe). This large clitoral structure is stimulated by vaginal thrusting, which also causes the swelling of the spongy erectile tissue in the front (anterior) wall of the vagina, in an area sometimes called the 'urethral sponge' or female prostate. This spongy area contains many tiny glands which can produce a fluid similar to the male prostatic fluid—thought to be the source of female 'ejaculation'. When this area fills with blood during sexual arousal, it can sometimes be felt through the vaginal wall—that's the G spot.[19]

Some of these areas have their own nervous pathways to the brain, according to Beverly Whipple from Rutgers University in New Jersey, who hit the news in the early 1970s writing about the G spot. Recently, Whipple, along with psychobiology professor Barry Komisaruk, has been tracking brain activity during sexual stimulation, testing reports from women with severely injured spines that they could still reach orgasm. How was this possible if their spinal cords were severed, cutting off the clitoral pathways to the brain?

What Whipple and Komisaruk found was a new nerve pathway which provided the sensory stimulus for orgasm. While most genital nerves connect to the brain via the spinal cord, the stimulation of areas deep in the vagina, including the cervix, connects with the brain by a different pathway—namely the vagus nerve, which winds from the brain through to the genitals, bypassing the spinal cord. It's this different connection which seems to allow many spinal cord–injured women to enjoy sexual pleasure. And for women who respond during thrusting, this may be part of their story.[20]

While women should be encouraged to feel comfortable about needing clitoral stimulation, it also makes sense for women not to ignore the delights that a vagina may have to offer—pleasures that some women learn only later in life, as Belinda (aged thirty-five) explains:

> I used to have a really hard time trying to come during sex (intercourse). But then it all changed. I'll never know what it was … a new partner with a different shaped penis, a very emotional time of my life, having had a baby, who knows? In my mid-thirties I suddenly starting coming during screwing. I now can come in most positions—with side-on 'scissor' positions particularly good. I often come just after my partner enters me and keep coming. He's a real athlete and able to put off his orgasm for as long as he likes (in fact sometimes can't get there at all!) but reads me perfectly and knows just how to move to keep me hovering, coming again and again.

Catherine Blackledge believes that many women just assume this won't happen for them. 'Our culture has kept the vagina from us. I get so angry when I keep reading in articles that the vagina is insensitive because the research clearly shows it is anything but that', she says. Blackledge believes the problem is also exacerbated by the way in which intercourse is portrayed in movies, particularly porn movies—'all that quick thrusting. Quick thrusting can be great but you need a balance. To experience vaginal orgasm you need to slow down so you can think and feel deep into these vaginal sensations. You need slow grinding, squeezing, and for the woman to use her vaginal muscles'.[21]

For a scientist, Blackledge is refreshingly willing to get personal. On the telephone from her office in London, she cheerfully discusses the first time she reached vaginal orgasm—with her fourth lover, a man with whom she felt safe and extremely comfortable—and the differences in her response to vaginal and direct clitoral stimulation.

But the very notion that some women *learn* to experience vaginal orgasms will be greeted by a shudder from therapists who've worked hard to convince women to relax and enjoy clitoral orgasms. They are rightly nervous that we might see a return to the old Freudian idea that women achieve sexual maturity by switching focus from the clitoris to the vagina. Freud argued that 'frigid' women fail to make the 'transfer of sensitivity' from the clitoral stimulation they experience in masturbation to responding to the vagina, mainly because they are paying too much attention to their clitorises. The role of the clitoris should be to set alight the vagina, he said, like 'pine shavings can be kindled to set a log of harder wood on fire'.[22]

His views were taken very seriously, particularly by his disciples. Freud's writings mention that Maria Bonaparte, leader of the psychoanalytic movement in France, twice had surgery to reposition her clitoral glans in an unsuccessful attempt to get the log burning. (Mary Roach, in her book *Bonk*, reports that while the clitoral repositioning procedure did nothing for Bonaparte, it was a success for two of her patients.)[23]

Heaven forbid that we buy into that judgemental frigidity talk. Yet why some women climax vaginally and others don't is an intriguing research question, one which has attracted the attention of Stuart Brody, a US psychology professor now working in Scotland. With his colleagues Ellen Laan and Rik Van Lunsen from the University of Amsterdam, he published research which sheds new light on one of the hot puzzles in current sex research.[24]

In Chapter 4, I talked about Pfizer's announcement that they were giving up on the search for pink Viagra. The reason was that while their research showed Viagra did increase pelvic blood flow—one of the physiological signs of arousal—many women didn't even notice. Well, Brody and colleagues wondered whether women who climax regularly in intercourse are more likely to make this connection, since pelvic blood flow is usually measured in the vagina. These European researchers had no trouble finding a large group of volunteer post-menopausal women who said they climaxed during intercourse (38 per cent claimed this happened every single time, and another 30 per cent most of or half the time). In the experiment, the women had their vaginal blood flow measured while being shown erotic videotapes. The scientists found that women who reported they didn't climax in intercourse were less likely than the coitally orgasmic women to show a correlation between vaginal blood flow and their subjective perception of arousal.

'For a woman to have an orgasm from intercourse, she has to be aware of and sensitive to erotic stimulation of her vagina. Unfortunately many women are not', comments Brody. He speculates that there may be a range of reasons why some women have this awareness and others not; these include physical sensitivity; different nerve pathways to the brain from the vagina and clitoris; having a skilled lover; issues of anatomical fit, such as the size and shape of the penis; and attention to sensations and appreciation of having a vagina. Brody also adds to the list: 'not being indoctrinated by anti-intercourse propaganda'.[25]

It now seems clear that many more women climax during intercourse than Shere Hite's proposed 30 per cent. (Hite was talking about women who climaxed in intercourse with 'no hands'—without adding extra clitoral stimulation.) And there is other data supporting this quite different picture. Even Kinsey, back in the 1950s, reported that more than half of his subjects reached orgasm in intercourse over 90 per cent of the time.[26] More recently, large surveys in both the UK and Australia have found that about 85 per cent of women report having had an orgasm during intercourse, with about half saying they climax this way most of the time. These latest studies involved twins—over 3000 of them in the Australian research—and aimed to find out whether genes influence women's ability to climax during intercourse. The answer was a resounding 'yes', with almost a third of the variation between women in their ability to climax during intercourse being due to genetic influences.[27]

That's really intriguing and has led to new work being done with twins, looking at whether women who climax during intercourse have different personalities from those who don't. Professor Nick Martin, from the Queensland Institute of Medical Research, heads up the group that conducted the Australian twins research. He reports that some of the parallel research from Britain has identified personality differences: 'Twins who rarely reach coital orgasm tend to be more introverted and less emotionally stable than the twins who do respond this way'.[28]

This research really would be valuable if it made it easier for women to enjoy a greater range of pleasure, including vaginal orgasms. But there's a very real risk that it may end up making those women who are currently content with their clitoral orgasms feel inadequate—and that would be turning back the clock in a most unhelpful way.

But it is important to recognise that there are plenty of women who do still enjoy penile thrusting, and that means it really does matter if men can't last long enough. What's long enough, you may ask. Penn State University researchers surveyed US and Canadian sex therapists to find out how long they thought intercourse should last—these experts suggested that less than three minutes was too short, and more than thirteen minutes was too long.[29]

What nonsense is this? Surely the important thing is that the man has some control over ejaculation so that he can prolong intercourse if that's what his partner prefers. Lead researcher Dr Eric Corty said that his study was 'designed to help calm couples' unrealistic beliefs that healthy sex should last for hours'.[30] Fair enough, but while I heard from many female diarists who'd be delighted if a shag came in under three minutes, I also heard from others who did sometimes enjoy making love for prolonged periods. Yes, even hours, provided they had occasional breaks to draw breath.

And I had some very cranky women who found themselves missing out because their partners lacked that control, like Barbara (aged fifty-eight) from Dubbo, who has been married to James for thirty-nine years:

> He's got a medical condition and is on strong medication. I think it causes erection problems—he won't speak to his doctor about it. And for a long time he's been experiencing premature ejaculation. I get disappointed and think, 'Buggar it. I can't be bothered even trying'. It makes me feel really crabby if I've really tried and am halfway there. Most likely this is why I don't even want to participate in the first place.

What a shame he won't speak to his doctor, because finally we are getting somewhere with this type of problem. Many men are able to teach themselves to last longer by using self-help sex therapy books which describe basic approaches—the squeeze technique, the stop–start technique, use of the pelvic muscles.

Bob (aged fifty-three) from Hobart tells an intriguing story. Here was a man who felt his sex life was reasonable but could have been better: 'I often felt I wasn't satisfying Jan properly'. About five years ago he came across an ad offering to improve the reader's sex life. He responded and ended up meeting a couple who told him all about multiple orgasms and how men can achieve them:

> The wife of the couple took me into a massage room, gave me a massage and then masturbated me, showing me how to control myself. It was amazing how well it worked. I went back about three more times and went from coming in about three to four minutes to about twenty-five to forty minutes. This certainly helped things at home.

The *Sex in Australia* survey found that about a quarter of men in all age groups reported 'coming too quickly'.[31] Some of these men wrestle with the problem all their lives. Researchers have discovered that ejaculation is controlled by serotonin receptors in the brain, and it appears that these men suffer from what may well be an inherited problem related to the sensitivity of these receptors—they simply have their ejaculatory threshold genetically set at a lower point, which results in them being more trigger-happy. Drug therapy that acts on these receptors is proving very effective in slowing these guys down. Low doses of anti-depressant drugs such as Zoloft or Aropax can work wonders, but these need to be taken continually to achieve the best results. Work is now underway on drugs which will be similarly effective when taken on demand, just before sex.

The frustrations of living with a trigger-happy man, however, are nothing compared to coping with the nasty sexual habits displayed by some of my male diarists. What really blew me away when reading some of the diaries were the men who simply refuse to get it, who don't understand the basics of what making love is all about. Read these stories and cringe!

> I was woken in the early morning with my nipples being milked like a cow, which hurts. (Carmen, forty-four)

> 6.20 a.m. this morning I was awoken from my sleep with Frank grabbing and pinching my nipples. Then, feeling it was sufficient, he started pushing his finger into my vagina enough to lubricate, then pulled me over and started pumping away with a half-erect penis. I said, 'Give me another half hour'. 'What?' he said, totally engrossed. I told him to stop—which he did. He got up angrily and went to the toilet. Within five minutes of getting back into the bed he went through the same repeat procedure, this time with fully erect penis. (Pat, forty-six)

> I asked him to touch my breasts while we were having sex in that position and he did but he was sort of squeezing them, wrenching them. I told him it wasn't doing much for me and he got cranky saying 'I can't touch your breasts and support myself' but he's done what I wanted plenty of times before. (Claire, thirty-two)

> Trev came to bed. I was drowsy. I kept to myself but his hand came creeping over. He did a really annoying thing—just a couple of fingers rubbing about an inch up and down on my arm, leg and side. Does he think that is going to turn me on? It is really irritating. He has been doing it for years. (Sally, forty-six)

> Sex is over-rated. It is sad to say I cannot remember when we had great sex. Most of the time it is over before I even get warmed up and most times he is asleep shortly after so I lie there and think of what just happened. I am over the

wham-bam-thank-you-mam sex. At times I feel, 'Why bother?' I'm over being disappointed. I have tried talking to him but it goes in one ear and out the other. I would like to have an amazing sex life, but have yet to find that. (Cath, fifty-one)

He has this thing about playing with my nipples. He knows I hate it and every time he does it, I threaten to put a bra on or slap him or really sulk and cry and then leave the bed. On Wednesday he wanted sex. He kissed me and stroked me so I turned over and kissed him back and then we finished off. I decided to have sex that time because I thought it might relax him, stop him from annoying me. Then last night he started pinching my nipples again. I asked him to stop, several times, but he wouldn't listen. I whacked him with the pillow and he seemed to get insulted and rolled over. I told him I would sleep in the study, told him if he wanted me back in bed he would have to apologise for being mean and nasty or ask me back. He didn't. I cried for a while but nothing. I finally slept. (Sophie, twenty)

There's a good reason why there are so many jokes about men being poor lovers, such as these:

Q. *What's the difference between a G spot and a golf ball?*
A. *A man will spend twenty minutes looking for a golf ball.*

Q. *Why don't women blink during foreplay?*
A. *They don't have time.*

Men's ineptitude and indifference to women's pleasure remains part of the problem when it comes to a female's lack of interest in sex. But after thirty-plus years of listening to men talking about sex, I have found that most men are desperately keen to go to bed with willing women and will do whatever they can to please them, however fumbling their efforts may be.

Of course, there are also cruel women, those who reject their partners in the most unfeeling manner, who laugh at and degrade them, or who refuse to pleasure them in the way they need. Luke complains that his erections aren't as easy as they used to be. 'When I was young I walked around with a stiffy for most of any given day', he says, but now he needs a helping hand. And despite the effort he has put into pleasuring his partner in just the way she likes, he finds that 'now when the shoe seems to be on the other foot, there is a reluctance or ignorance to return the favour so to speak'.

Yet the strongest complaint from men had nothing to do with their own pleasure. What they wanted, what they yearned for, was for women to share their secrets, their desires. 'Women simply won't do it', complains Ivan. Here he is talking about his partner, Suzie:

> I spent years trying to work out what she liked and what turned her on. This is a woman who has real trouble talking about sex and whose main method of communication is a whispered yes, a small groan, a tensing of her leg muscles, so it was a difficult process.

Then one day, Ivan wrote to me, so excited. He had had a breakthrough!

> We got to the dressing room. Did she want a creaming? Yes, she did. I warmed the moisturiser. There was a time when she would let me undress her. Not now. Scurry into bed. Complain about the cold. Defer the action until she's warm enough and ready enough. But we embraced; lying on our sides, facing each other, eyes open, and I held her and, of course, couldn't refrain from stroking. This apparently had appeal and the stroking became more sensual, in the course of which she told me to spend more time on her breasts, but very lightly. Along the way, she said, 'Not so firm, do it more gently'. 'Less attention to the

nipples.' 'Stroke all of the breast.' So then I put moisturiser on my hand, which enabled me to smoothly and lightly cup my hand under her breast and run my fingers here and there. And all the while I was thinking, 'Suzie is actually communicating! She's telling me what she wants me to do! Hallelujah!'

Ivan is seventy-four years old. He has been making love to Suzie for thirty-five years.

Men's quest to explore their lovers' minds is immensely moving. They write so eloquently about wanting to know her, wanting to share her secrets and their intense frustration at being shut out.

Here's Sam, from Brisbane: 'How many women do you know who will let their man wander around in their heads, who will not only let him peek into the closets of their minds but will slide open the drawers, so he can see? Am I a freak for wanting this?' He explains his frustration at trying to persuade his loving wife to be more open with him:

> Sometimes I find it difficult to know the difference between a sound that means 'Ouch' and one that means 'Yesssss ... more!' It can be frustrating and it can lead to clumsiness on my part as I search to discover what works and what does not on any particular occasion.

Intimacy is not for the faint of heart, writes David Schnarch in his wonderful book *Passionate Marriage*. He's one of the few therapists writing about sex who talks about helping couples to achieve a deeper emotional connection—'I know your essence and you know me'. He knows what these men yearn for. Read his descriptions of sex where couples look deeply into each other's eyes as they climax, his talk of 'fucking, doing and being done', a partner's face 'melting'—all the intensely erotic experiences that take sex to a different emotional plane. Schnarch so rightly concludes that exploring the limits of sexual potential has little to do with clever techniques but a lot to do with how two people feel about themselves and each other outside the bedroom. It's these personal and interpersonal issues—feelings of shame, embarrassment, lack of confidence in oneself and one's partner—that stand in the way of achieving that potential.[32]

What a treat it is to find couples who have that connection, who know all about the 'wall-socket sex' presented by Schnarch as an ideal—that all-consuming mutual desire, heart-stopping intimacy and deep personal meaningfulness. They are truly the lucky ones.

12

It's in His Kiss!
That's Where It Is

What is it about the kiss? That's what many women really crave. Women who feel lonely in their marriages often long for those passionate, knee-trembling smooches they once shared with their lovers—hours spent in each other's arms, nibbling, kissing, lips moving, tongues touching.

Women talk about the yearning they feel as they watch young lovers embracing in the park. They find it almost unbearable to sit in the movies, watching their favourite movie stars gazing longingly into each other's eyes, moving closer, his hand gently stroking her neck, tilting his head until their lips gently meet. That's what many women tell me they miss most.

'Finding out that I wasn't going to be able to have a great pash with my husband was one of the saddest realisations I have ever had', says Claire, a 32-year-old Sydney woman. She regards herself as happily married but would prefer a lot more sex than what she's getting, and is frustrated by a lack of variety in lovemaking. What she really longs for, though, is the kiss:

> I'd really love to have a relationship where kissing passionately was something that stood alone in the relationship—not just part of sex. When Geoff kisses me during sex I feel like he is just going through the motions because he doesn't want to do it any other time. I'd love to be with someone who wanted to

kiss me passionately during the course of the day. I fantasise about being with a mythical soul mate who'd scoop me up in a passionate embrace in the middle of the kitchen.

It isn't only that they never kiss passionately when they are not in bed. She's also unhappy about the way her husband, Geoff, does it:

> I just LURVE a good pash, locked lips, tongues sliding over the top of each other. Mmmm. I tried to coach him on this earlier in the relationship without success. I have been told that I am a very good kisser, and most guys seem to follow my lead on kissing style and get the hang of it even if they aren't that good to begin with. They allow themselves to be educated but not Geoff. He just keeps doing what he's always done. Kissing is such a turn on for me. When I was with my first boyfriend and our sexual interactions were quite innocent, I would often come just kissing, provided I was sitting on him, or him lying on top of me, putting pressure on my clit.

As Claire's diaries reveal, she does try to teach Geoff but he never seems to get it right:

> Last night when I got into bed, Geoff was up for a bit. He was trying to please me, and he was asking me what I liked. I asked him to kiss me. He doesn't like kissing—he says that I am stealing his air. He tried, but *sigh*, he is just a terrible kisser. If we are just kissing each other lightly on the lips, it's OK, but after a little of that I want more passion. If we are using tongues, he puts his whole mouth over the top of mine so I feel like I am kissing inside of his mouth, and there is no lip-to-lip contact if he is using his tongue. I can still remember kisses from years back that knocked me off my feet. The best ones were the first kisses with a new partner, where there was a delicious tension just before the kiss. In my fantasies there is always a pause to drink in that moment; it often saddens me that real life doesn't play out like that any more.

With so many women complaining about how their partners kiss, you wonder if they always felt like that or whether during the heady, romantic early days of their relationships, any deficiencies in technique were swamped by the chemical high.

Phoebe (aged thirty-six) from Melbourne tells me that kissing —the long, romantic, perfect kiss—features a lot in her fantasies and dreams, while the enjoyment she gets from kissing her husband is decreasing:

> In fact, I don't think Larry was ever the best kisser but previously, high hormones and excitement had masked it. Now the desire for a real kiss is haunting me. It feels like a return of an idealistic and maybe even sacred desire. I just don't really feel that into him very often. And I don't really like kissing him on the lips much either, which I could take as some terrible sign that it's all over but which I prefer to see just as a sign that things have changed since I was twenty-four.

When that glorious, romantic, 'in love' stage known as limerence is over, we drop the rose-coloured glasses. A man's poor kissing technique is starkly revealed in the harsh glare of a normal, flawed relationship, when women may focus only on what he does wrong. The following assortment of diary entries testifies to this:

> I have to tell you this—I really don't enjoy kissing with him. He has no lips and when he tries to get passionate, they are just hard little lines. Horrible, not his fault I know. So basically he kisses with his face, I suppose, is the best way to describe it, and that is usually prickly. Often feels like kissing a pin cushion with the wrong ends sticking out. Another thing that used to drive me insane was that whenever he kissed me he had to finish with the loud 'breaking the suction' kiss noise. Ahhhhhhhhhh. Eventually I said something and he doesn't do that any more. Am I just a bitch or is he really clueless?

I have never enjoyed kissing my husband. Sad but true. I find it repulsive—always have. This has been a matter of regret for him. The chemistry has always been totally wrong. I have dodged kissing him for most of the time we were together and I don't think he has ever understood why! But I used to like kissing—especially in the pre-sex days.

Another thing I've noticed: I can't stand the sound his mouth makes just before he kisses me—kind of a sticky, sucky sound … I can't bear to bring it up just yet; I don't think he's over the time I told him he didn't brush his teeth enough (although that didn't make him brush them any more often—maybe I should try to be more tactful!).

He doesn't know how to kiss. Hasn't been to the dentist since I've known him—twenty-four years. I started to think, 'Yuk'. I don't know how to tell him. It would crush him.

I hate kissing now and I used to LOVE it. We kissed all the time and now it repulses me. I can't tell him that because it would really hurt him. I use so many excuses: he hasn't brushed his teeth, he hasn't shaved. I don't get turned on with kissing any more and it used to make me have a pit in my stomach.

Women use kissing as a mate-assessment device, says Gordon Gallup, an evolutionary psychologist at the State University of New York in Albany. He argues that kissing involves a very complicated exchange of information—olfactory, tactile and 'postural adjustments' that tap into underlying mechanisms (both evolved and unconscious) that enable women to make determinations about their partners. 'Once in a committed relationship women use kissing to update and monitor the status of their relationship with their partner', he suggests. 'They are attempting to assess and carefully evaluate potential changes in their relationship and

their partner's commitment to that relationship.' Gallup reports
there is evidence that the amount of kissing between partners is
directly related to relationship satisfaction.[1]

Loretta (aged forty-four) from Brisbane has always adored kissing: 'I find it very erotic. My ex-husband hated long, deep, passionate kissing. He didn't mind a quick peck, but nothing else'.
But then she met John, who also loves kissing:

> His ex-wife hated kissing as well which frustrated and disap-
> pointed him. So when we started going out together it was like
> a kisser's dream come true for us. Kissing in a deep, passionate
> and intimate way is the quickest way to get me into the mood.
> It is an absolute must in any long-term relationship.

So there are men who are into kissing, some of whom also
find themselves with partners who aren't interested in it. David
(aged sixty-six) from Melbourne was surprised to find that his
wife, Margaret (aged sixty-three), has gone off the activity: 'I'd be
happy to use my mouth in any pleasurable way. But for Marg it
doesn't seem to engage much. I'm sad that our kissing lacks the
passion that I'd like to express. I think Marg would feel suffocated
if I expressed myself as I used to'.

To make matters worse, he once fancied himself as a good
kisser: 'Pre-marriage, women told me I kissed as well as anybody,
so I feel like a talent has gone to waste!' And he says that his wife
is also not much into other oral activity:

> Marg accepts oral sex from me occasionally. She associates
> getting thrush with oral sex so likes to limit it, but she enjoys
> it when it occurs. I think Marg has given me oral sex on three
> occasions! It's just not a pleasure for her so I don't push it.

Margaret admits she doesn't like kissing any more. 'Before I
was married I did want to kiss Dave—long and hard. I don't know
when I stopped liking it. I suspect it was when I no longer wanted

to give myself lock, stock and barrel to him', she says, explaining the struggle early in their marriage over her sense that he didn't really accept her as she was. Kissing came to represent giving in: 'It symbolised giving up the real me'. But now the couple have moved on to a new level of intimacy and Margaret is pondering whether her desire for kissing might come back:

> As I've got closer to Dave these last years, I have initiated kissing him on the head, face, neck, body, even lips. But not kissing where the tongue and saliva are mixed. I think that maybe I'm getting closer to that. But not yet. I'm interested to see if I can ever kiss the old way again.

The last word in this chapter on kissing comes from an intriguing source. Gay (thirty-six) used to be a sex worker but now works in Alice Springs as a nurse. When she first wrote to me, she was three months in to a passionate live-in relationship with Bart (aged forty), a former jockey. She's the first to admit that they are an unlikely couple: 'He is very lightweight and toned and muscled where I am obese and not very healthy at all. I am nearly double his weight, and we are about the same height. I am 100 kilograms and he is around 60 kilograms'.

But this small man knows all about pleasing women. For a start, he's multi-orgasmic. The forty pages of diaries that Gay wrote for me included details of numerous days where they made love two or three times, with Bart enjoying up to five ejaculations and Gay having the time of her life. She is a very sexually experienced woman but he was the first to get her to climax in intercourse—just one of his many talents. 'I think many women in this world would have a hugely increased sex drive if they had a taste of my man', she boasts. He's also a man who loves kissing, says Gay:

> The very first thing that Bart did when we got into bed together for the first time was kiss me passionately. He seems to kiss

with his whole body. He knows kissing drives me wild and he makes sure he does it plenty. He is so soft and passionate when he touches me, there are deep kisses, long touches, he plays with my hair and puts his hands gently on my face and neck while he is kissing me. He kisses during sex and responds well to my movements and wants. He loves to make me orgasm and will often hold back on his own because he wants to give me another one. That is what makes his sex so good to me. He is hard and fast when he wants to be, but with foreplay he is sooo gentle.

This woman, who knows so much about pleasing men, is now on the receiving end—her diaries make such sexy reading. She's very well placed to offer some words of wisdom.

Don't forget kissing, she tells everybody. 'I think kissing should be done both in the sex act and out of the bedroom. If I am stressed or upset, Bart knows to grab me and give me a deep kiss and it will relax me instantly.' This wordly woman warns that the kiss is often one of the first things to go in a relationship:

> I think sometimes if men were to pay more attention to the kiss at times other than in bed, a woman might feel more attractive and wanted. If there is a kiss that is unconditional—just to say 'I love you'—it might make the woman feel more loved and worthy of attention. Then she may be more willing to give a bit more in the bedroom.

Of course, this is nothing new. 'It's in his kiss', sang a 22-year-old Aretha Franklin back in 1964. And she was right. That is just where it is.

13

Three Cheers for Mr Pinocchio

Many years ago I was driving past a newsagency when I glanced over and received a huge shock. Outside the shop was a newspaper billboard with the massive headline 'BETTINA ARNDT— I WAS WRONG ABOUT SEX!'

What on earth was this? It must have been a slow news day because the paper was beating up an interview I'd just given on the previous decade of sex research. This was the early 1980s and we were finally beginning to discover a little more about the mysteries of erections. I had shared with a journalist my guilt about spending years as a sex therapist reassuring men that their erectile problems were all in their mind, that they were due purely to anxiety. Now sex researchers were finding out that we were wrong—it was their bodies that were letting them down. Erectile dysfunction was emerging mainly as a physical problem, with blood flow difficulties at the heart of men's failure to stand to attention.

That was good news and bad. Yes, it was a blow to discover it wasn't simply a matter of persuading men to calm down, take it easy and let nature take its course. But at least we knew there was a good reason why this wasn't working for many of the men we were seeing. No amount of relaxation exercises or gentle, graduated approaches to intercourse would help a man recover his potency if his plumbing had broken down.

Soon after this, we gained miracle drugs which promised erections even to men who had been sexual cripples for many years. When Viagra burst onto the scene, I was delighted. I thought about all those men who'd come to see me, those who had choked back tears as they had described the devastating impact of their lost erections. They had taught me to understand how much it matters to them. Impotence cuts men to the quick. It represents such a loss to their sense of selves, their sense of manhood. But rarely do we acknowledge what they are experiencing.

Rob from Perth was very restrained when he first volunteered for my research. The sixty-five year old described his long, loving marriage and the very active sex life he had until four years ago, when he discovered he had prostate cancer. The cancer was successfully removed but he's been left partially impotent. His wife, Jenny, has been wonderfully supportive:

> I remember that before the operation she said that we needed to make love as much as possible as things would never be the same. We made love every day for those few weeks. I did not believe her at the time, but she was right (as she most always is) and I have not had a proper erection since. I have found it very difficult to adjust to this, but with experimentation and patience we again have a satisfactory sex life, although it will never be quite the same as it once was. The spontaneity is missing and the days of my curling up behind Jenny and being inside her as we go to sleep are no longer possible. We miss that.

I wrote back to him, saying I understood what a blow that must be to him. I told him I have always thought that erections are the most wonderful things, so it isn't surprising that men miss them terribly if they no longer happen. Months later, after writing diaries for me and corresponding, he confessed he'd been feeling mighty low when he'd first made contact, and how much it had helped to have someone acknowledge his loss:

I think I had been feeling sorry for myself, possibly a bit depressed about it and initially feeling I was no longer a whole man. For some reason that I cannot explain, just being in contact with you has made me think things through and I feel much better about my situation. I feel at peace now and appreciate that the ways Jenny and I have found together to pleasure each other and to both have orgasms is just so wonderful, that I am content and am really very happy with our sex lives. To me, pleasuring Jenny and bringing her to orgasm is so very satisfying and gives me mountains of pleasure. If I come too, then that is a bonus.

A chance remark can make such a difference. How sad that we rarely treat this issue seriously. Think about the reaction when Viagra came on sale—the endless quips, the silly chatter. A man's loss of erections is so often seen as a joke. Our drug regulators decided there was no need for the public subsidisation of treatments for impotence—these are 'lifestyle' drugs, they sneered. That is very different from the respect we pay to women's relationship to their bodies and their sexuality. When a woman has a mastectomy, we are naturally solicitous about the impact this will have on her confidence as a woman. Her need for breast reconstruction is totally accepted and understood. Yet when the legacy of cancer is a limp penis rather than a lost breast, all we do is giggle and snicker.

Rob was one of the unlucky ones, with the damage from his cancer operation too great even for the new wonder drugs to work. He's tried Caverject injections, Cialis and Viagra: 'I was allergic to the injections—the drug caused such a painful erection I could hardly bear to have my glans touched. The tablets had no effect except to make me feel poorly, with headaches and a hot, red face'. He'd had a 'nerve sparing' operation but his urologist told him these procedures often cause massive nerve and blood vessel damage, and that some patients are luckier than others with respect to potency. Rob says:

> If the penis is a barometer of man's readiness for sex, mine has busted. Not even watching an X-rated movie causes any penile stirrings, although mentally I am stirred. The only thing that will cause any increase in size is manual stimulation of the glans area by Jenny or me, but erection is only about 50 per cent of what it used to be.

However, this is an inventive man who has worked hard to overcome the obstacles to lovemaking. His beloved wife, Jenny, has always enjoyed penetration—she usually comes during inter-course—but her main orgasm tends to happen when she's lying on top of him. With experimentation, they found that this still works with the right pressure on the clitoris, even without his erection. 'We then discovered that once she was aroused from foreplay, if she lay on top of me with my limp penis against her clitoris, with some thrusting movements she would have an orgasm and sometimes I would too', says Rob. But he felt that her orgasm could be improved 'if she had something thrusting into her vagina'.

Enter Mr Pinocchio. That's what the couple call the 'artificial penis' Rob bought in a sex shop, to which he has added his own improvisation:

> I found a way to make this 'prosthesis' work as my penis. I have a piece of foam rubber and have cut a hole in it so that the bottom end of Mr P fits into it. I hold this between my crossed thighs and it extends up over my balls, ready for penetration, suitably lubricated. When Jenny is ready, she lies over me, inserts Mr P and places my glans against her clitoris. With my legs I then thrust gently into her and it is very similar to the real thing. This results in orgasm, sometimes for both of us, and is very satisfying.

Three cheers for Mr Pinocchio!

It is so great that this couple has discovered a way to regain much of the pleasure they had always shared together. But I heard from many other couples who found that the new drugs worked beautifully. Remember Michael and Heather, the Adelaide couple with the calendars and nightly underwear parade from Chapter 2? Michael started using Levitra when he began having trouble with his erections and found that the drug also helped him to delay ejaculation:

> I was about sixty-four when I noticed my erections weren't so firm so I started taking a small dose of Levitra, which not only helped my erections but to my surprise I found I was lasting longer, which was a real bonus. The only downside for me is a mild headache and I have to anticipate action because it absorbs better if taken before meals and without alcohol.

Mr Pinocchio Isn't the Only Answer

For men who are having trouble standing to attention, there is now a range of options which may help. There have been great advances in the treatment of erectile problems in the past ten years or so. You need to get over your embarrassment and go to your local doctor to find out what is best for you—don't get sucked in by private clinics who offer anonymity in return for the payment of large sums of money for treatments that probably won't work. Here, in brief, are the main proven treatments:

Tablets

Viagra (sildenafil) was the first tablet on sale for erectile dysfunction and remains the best known of the phosphodiesterase type 5 (PDE5) inhibitors. Cialis (tadalafil) and Levitra (vardenafil) are similar medications. They all work by inhibiting a particular enzyme in the penis, increasing blood flow and enhancing erectile response to normal sexual stimulation. There's little difference in the effectiveness of the three drugs—they all take about an hour to kick in—but with Cialis, the effect lasts much longer: thirty-six hours compared with up to twelve for the other two drugs. A high-fat meal makes Viagra and Levitra slower to absorb. For the best results, it is also advisable to limit alcohol intake to two drinks when taking these medications; intoxication makes them less effective.

These drugs are not aphrodisiacs. They do not make a man want to have sex, but merely help his sexual plumbing to work normally, provided he is sexually stimulated. The medication works successfully in about 65 to 70 per cent of men with erectile problems and results in about 80 per cent of full penile rigidity.

Directions for beginning treatment with these tablets include the following:

- Begin with the maximum dose unless there are medical reasons not to do this.
- Wait one hour after dosing before attempting intercourse.
- Engage in direct stimulation of the penis to maximise erection.
- Limit alcohol to two drinks before sex.
- Take Viagra and Levitra on an empty stomach the first few times.
- Before you decide that these tablets don't work for you, make sure you take at least six to eight doses.

Once these tablets are working, the dose can be reduced, intercourse may be attempted sooner after taking the medication, and they can all be taken with food.

Side effects occur in about one in ten men and can include headaches, facial flushing, indigestion and nasal congestion. A small percentage of men develop a blue-green tinge to their vision with Viagra and Levitra, while lower back and thigh pain can occur with Cialis. After repeated doses, the side effects tend to diminish. These drugs are not suitable for men who are not fit enough to engage in sex due to cardiovascular disease, men who are taking medicines containing nitrates for the treatment of angina (heart pain) or men who use amyl nitrate 'poppers' recreationally.

Penile Injections

Before the arrival of the Viagra-like drugs, Caverject injection therapy was the most popular and effective treatment. It involves the man or his partner using a very fine needle to inject alprostadil (also known as prostaglandin E-1) into the penis. This drug relaxes the penile blood vessels, allowing them to expand. It can create an erection within five to ten minutes that lasts up to an hour. This therapy works whether the penis is stimulated or not, and often results in a more rigid erection than that produced by the PDE5 inhibitors. Caverject should not be used more than once in a 24-hour period and not more than three times a week.

This treatment requires some dexterity, good eyesight and a little practice to learn the technique; an automatic injection device is also available. Men with certain illnesses, such as leukaemia, multiple myeloma and sickle-cell anaemia, should not use this drug. Possible side effects include a temporary burning pain after injection, bruising at the injection site, scarring of the tissues of the penis after repeated injections and a prolonged erection lasting four hours or more. However, many men have used these injections successfully and safely for many years.

Devices

Vacuum devices consist of an airtight cylinder, pump and ring. The cylinder is placed over the lubricated flaccid penis. A hand-held or battery-operated pump is used to push air out of the cylinder, creating a vacuum which draws blood into the penis. When the penis is erect, a rubber ring is slid off the end of the tube and onto the base of the penis to keep the blood from flowing out. (The ring comes in different sizes.)

When intercourse is finished, the ring is taken off and the penis goes down—after thirty minutes, the ring must be removed or the penis can be damaged.

Vacuum erection devices are generally effective and safe, and can be used as often as needed. Side effects can include penile bruising, coldness, numbness and a bluish tinge to the penis. Some practice is usually needed to master this device.

Penile rings on their own are suitable for men who can create an erection but not maintain it. They are placed around the base of the penis, helping it to stay erect enough for intercourse. Some men take a PDE5 inhibitor tablet as well as using a vacuum device with a ring, or they use a ring on its own.

Ivan (aged seventy-three) had an operation for an enlarged prostate ten years ago. Afterwards, he could still reach orgasm but ceased to ejaculate—that wasn't a big deal—but then he started having erectile difficulties. 'This became a problem for me and, although she denied it, a problem for my wife. Our relationship began to deteriorate. My doctor prescribed Viagra. I used half a tablet at a time. Immediately effective. Our relationship improved', he writes, adding that the only hitch now is that Viagra needs an hour in his system to take effect, which detracts from spontaneity. But he's managing fine.

'There is really nothing worse than wanting to have sex but not being able to maintain an erection. It's very disappointing for both parties and soul-destroying for a man. Gone is what makes you a man'—this is Ted, from a mango farm in northern Queensland. The fifty-nine year old has had the occasional erection problem over the past twelve years or so: 'Initially I would find everything worked fine but during prolonged sex, that is if I didn't ejaculate in the first five to six minutes of intercourse, I would lose my erection. Any alcohol consumption at all seemed to magnify the problem'.

His doctor recommended injection therapy, which worked well, but then Viagra came onto the market and it worked a treat. More recently, Ted has switched to Cialis, 'which I find seems to last longer and is slightly more effective'. The cost was getting him down but he was lucky enough to stumble across a friendly chemist, a man close to his own age, who was using the same drug. 'Isn't it wonderful? This drug has breathed new life into my marriage and makes life worth living again', the chemist told him, encouraging him to get his doctor to order the highest dose of the drug and split them into four to six pieces, to get the cost right down. 'I currently take a quarter of a tablet every two to three days. Any longer between doses results in not maintaining an erection', says Ted.

So now everything is fine. Ted's libido remains at a healthy level—he and his wife, Rikki, have sex almost every night, sometimes during the night and in the mornings too. Rikki confesses that she's sometimes a little reluctant to initiate sex: 'I don't know if he has taken a tablet or not and I don't want to put him in a situation where he may not be able to respond'. But with Cialis lasting up to thirty-six hours, it's usually not a problem. Ted loves it when she makes a move: 'It shows me that I am desired, and I feel very lucky and spoilt. Women are not exclusive in their need to have reassurance that they are loved and desired'.

These drugs are a godsend, says Ted. And so they are—for many thousands of men across the world. That's why it is infuriating that there are still so many sharks out there who are determined to rip men off with shonky treatments that simply don't work. I was recently at a fathers' festival where I watched in fury as the owner of a natural health company sneered at Viagra, hugely exaggerating the drug's risks and side effects. He then flogged his 'natural' product, making nonsensical, pseudo-scientific claims about its effects on potency. All natural health products are now fully supported by scientific evidence, he claimed.

That is such hogwash. A minuscule 1 per cent of the altern- ative medicine sold in this country is actually assessed for quality, safety and efficacy by the Therapeutic Goods Administration (TGA), the body charged with regulating this industry. Yet a recent South Australian survey showed that it is widely believed by consumers that all such products are properly tested.[1] Most natural health products sold in Australia are simply 'listed' by the TGA, which means that the organisation usually has not even asked for the manufacturer's evidence that the product works or is safe. Yet these goods can still be advertised using 'low level' claims. So my snake oil salesman can get away with claiming on his product's labels that they 'maximise blood flow to where you need it most'—a claim which has no scientific proof.

How outrageous that this is still happening when men now have their golden fleece. Here we have a very good range of effective, proven impotence treatments that can help most of the men suffering from such problems; impotent men have never had it so good. But there's also a very determined shonky industry that is keen to muscle in on this lucrative market. In 2007, one of these unsavoury companies boasted that it had made a profit of over $22 million from the erectile dysfunction and premature ejaculation treatments offered in its clinics. That astonishing amount of money has been taken from vulnerable men who have been left struggling with faulty equipment, when medical science may well have the answer to their plight.

My anger about these companies and their clinics went up a few notches when I wrote about them in a newspaper column and received a legal threat. My 2007 Christmas week started with a letter from a top-flight law firm threatening to sue me for speaking out on this issue. The bully boys were at it again. Whenever anyone in the media talks about the massive rip-offs occurring in the impotence industry, the people who run the cashed-up clinics bring in the legal guns.

I'm sure you are aware of the advertisements on radio, television and in magazines across Australia for private clinics offering their unique treatments for impotence and premature ejaculation. Men who are too embarrassed to see their local doctor are flocking to them. But many of the operators in this dubious industry don't even offer men the proven, legitimate products as the first line of treatment. That's because these don't give the sharks enough of a mark-up. Instead, the clinics coerce men into shelling out hundreds, sometimes even thousands of dollars for products made of compounds of up to eight different drugs, often presented in a nasal spray, claiming that the combination of medication produces better results—that mythical stronga, longa donga.

What a lot of rubbish. It's like trying to make a soufflé by randomly throwing together assorted ingredients from half a dozen different recipes—the chances of it rising are very slim indeed. The problem is that if you tell impotent men that you are offering a whizzbang treatment, some will end up with erections even if you give them sugar water. Research shows that the placebo effect is very strong, particularly with psychological impotence. So the clinics do have some success stories. But what they don't have is properly conducted research proving that the particular combination of drugs they use actually works. Sure, they can produce graphs showing years of research on each of the drugs in their mix, but nothing to support their particular smorgasbords.

Our real medical experts are united in condemning these little cocktails as most likely ineffective, and possibly dangerous. In 1998, the New South Wales Government held an inquiry into impotence treatment services.[2] At the time, the main treatment that was available involved injection therapy, but here, too, clinics were profiteering by using expensive combinations of drugs rather than the ones that were proven to be safe and effective. In its report, the ministerial committee concluded that the multi-drug approach was scientifically dubious and recommended single-drug therapy as the first treatment option. But here we are, ten years later, and many of the same clinics are still at it, now combining drugs into nasal sprays which have never been proven to be effective in this form for the treatment of erection problems and premature ejaculation.

In 2003, these companies received another rap over the knuckles, this time by the Federal Court, which found that their clinics were engaging in misleading and deceptive conduct—lying about their guaranteed results, the medical safety of their treatments, the experience of their doctors and the side effects of their treatments, as well as bullying patients into long and expensive treatment contracts. Yet, four years later, the clinics operated by just one of these companies pulled in $22 million from these treatments.

The government needs to act to close the legal loophole that allows people to be exploited through combinations of legitimate drugs promoted as some magical super cure. But men also need to wake up and not allow themselves to be duped. Sure, it is embarrassing to front a GP and seek help in finding the drugs which might really work for you, but that's the only way to ensure you won't be exploited. You can obtain the name of local doctors specialising in this area from Impotence Australia (www. impotenceaustralia.com.au), a website supported by some of

Australia's real impotence experts, who can also help with premature ejaculation and other male sex problems. The government-sponsored website Andrology Australia (www.andrologyaustralia. org) will also give you accurate information about treatments. And don't sign contracts for any treatment—any legitimate practitioners will offer trial runs of the proven products, which are available by prescription. Clinics charging large sums of money for such treatments are usually offering a dubious product which is unlikely to work.

It was heart-breaking talking to people volunteering to write diaries who had already paid out hundreds of dollars for these useless treatments. When Brisbane woman Sheila (aged fifty-five) first wrote to me, she wasn't sure if she and her partner, Chris, would qualify for the research project because sex simply wasn't happening for them. Chris (aged sixty), whose lack of sex drive seemed linked to his problem with premature ejaculation, was awaiting the arrival of some new wonder drug he'd ordered through a newspaper advertisement. The couple had been together for only eighteen months.

Sheila told me she'd always had a strong libido: 'In fact, since menopause, I seem to be wanting sex more than ever'. Yet with Chris now, the sex is over almost as soon as they begin. 'When he does have an erection and we begin sex, it's over in seconds, with me missing out on an orgasm, so you can imagine how frustrating it is for me', says Sheila.

Chris had already forked out over $500 to one clinic for a nasal spray, which did nothing. Another $400 to $500 bought him the new wonder drug—it turned out to be some sort of testosterone cream, which proved equally useless. When I finally managed to speak to Chris to refer him to proper help, it was obvious how being so thoroughly ripped-off was adding to this vulnerable man's burden.

My conversations with Sheila brought home to me how tough these problems can be for the partner, who worries about her man's plight but also rightly feels somewhat deprived. It is very difficult for women to support their partners without adding to the pressure. What makes it particularly hard is that the men often retreat, avoiding sex, not wanting to talk about it. Problems like premature ejaculation or erectile dysfunction often underlie lost libido in men, as the man who loses confidence in his erectile ability or ejaculation control avoids performing when it carries the risk of failure.

With over half of all men over fifty experiencing erectile problems, that means huge numbers of older couples are struggling with these issues.[3] Add to these the men who have treatment for prostate cancer, many of whom subsequently have difficulty with erections.[4] However, now that this surgery is so common, we are seeing more open discussion of its impact, including the fallout in relationships.

Sharon's husband, Steve, had nerve-sparing surgery and ended up impotent. They tried Viagra, but got only a slight response. Here's Sharon writing on a website for men who are recovering from prostate surgery: 'As the months went on, his libido vanished, much to his distress and confusion. I felt that he had withdrawn from me and our 38-year marriage began to deteriorate because of the emotional non-intimacy, not because of my sexual frustration'.[5]

The more he withdrew the more anxious and upset she became:

> I don't suppose I ever feared Steve didn't love me any more, but I did feel he loved me like a 90-year-old lady. I even got mad and mean once and said that if I'd wanted a good roommate I wouldn't have chosen him! I wanted a husband.

They tried Caverject, the injection therapy, but it caused an 'ache' (a rare side effect of this drug is a temporary burning pain).

'It was hard for either of us to have pleasurable anticipation of a sexual event when we both knew the result would be hours of pain!' says Sharon. Steve's libido stayed low; his interest in using the injections was naturally minimal. 'My hurt at his emotional withdrawal was such that I wasn't sure I even wanted sex with him', she adds.

But then they had a breakthrough, discovering another injection drug that worked well. 'We rediscovered the joy of erections without pain. His libido has returned to normal. That first-ever threat to our marriage is certainly gone', Sharon writes. She advises other couples in this situation to tackle the problem rather than pretend it is not happening:

It's worth mourning, by BOTH of them. That's OK. What's not OK is for either one to pretend they don't care. Some men are more bothered than others, and quite often the women have been especially bothered by the man's apparent emotional withdrawal from all forms of intimacy.

Some of my diarists were tiptoeing through much the same territory. It was intriguing to see how careful the women were to avoid putting more pressure on their men. When impotence comes on top of a cancer scare, it's natural that a loving partner will be very nervous of doing anything to increase the man's anxiety.

Meg, from Brisbane, is the perfect example. Hers is a fascinating story. The fifty-six year old has been married to Paul for thirty-five years: 'We started going out together when I was eighteen, he was twenty-three. Don't laugh at the next bit. It's true. I was a virgin until I married. We came from deeply religious backgrounds and met through church activities'.

The two of them went on to become one of my most sexually active couples. Initially in their relationship, however, things weren't so great, as the contraceptive pill reduced Meg's drive and she was distracted by the demands of her career: 'Once the initial excitement wore off, I found myself looking for excuses not to have sex. I also had not experienced orgasm at that stage which was most disappointing. However we still had sex fairly regularly'.

They started a family, producing three children fairly quickly. Then came a crisis in their marriage. 'It was triggered by non-sexual issues, which could have very easily split us', says Meg. As they worked through the problem, Meg decided to act on the advice given to her in pre-marriage counselling by their minister —that men have a biological need for sex. 'I realised that it is best in a marriage to try and meet his needs', she says, adding that she still thinks of herself as a feminist but now believes in not saying 'no' unless she is genuinely too exhausted:

> Our sex lives improved and I started having orgasms which naturally meant I wanted a lot more sex. We decided to really set time aside to have sex and get a lock on the bedroom door. We had sex almost every night, sometimes twice and occasionally three times.

In their forties and fifties, their sex was fantastic, Meg says. 'It could not have been better in both quality and quantity.' They maintained that lively pace until just after her husband's sixtieth birthday, when he was diagnosed with prostate cancer. 'I had to try to keep both of our spirits up although I cried a lot thinking about what was going to happen to our sex life. Not only was it a source of much pleasure and joy, it was also a means of consolation for us', she says.

Fortunately, the surgery appears to have eradicated the cancer and the nerves that control erections were able to be spared, but, as Meg says, 'it has been a difficult road back'. They have tried the injections, which left Paul feeling numb, and Cialis caused tummy upsets. It took a while to regain spontaneous erections: 'Nine months after the operation, he woke up with an erection and away we went. Never miss an opportunity now and he's a lot happier'.

Since the operation, Meg doesn't climax during intercourse any more, mainly because his erections are less firm:

> He feels fairly sensitive about this, so I have to be careful. I have tried to reassure him that it doesn't matter at the end of the day. I'm grateful that the cancer has been eradicated and we can have sex unaided. I feel I have to put my needs on the back burner for a while. I just go with the flow and accept what happens. I feel pleasure for me will most probably be through self-stimulation—while I'm at it I think of the good past times and we've had plenty.

She even acknowledges there were times in the past when she thought they might have overdone the sex: 'I should have been up getting on with housework, but I stayed in bed. Now, of course, I have no regrets about that'.

Meg is thankful that her man is well and that intercourse has resumed, with regular masturbation also on the menu. Her diaries are brief but cheerful.

Saturday—Meg's diary

Usual early morning sex. Best for erections for someone of sixty-one who has had prostate cancer. Half-asleep when it all starts. In recent times our usual position is the scissors. I am flat on my back while he is on his side. Can relax after without moving—good for after-cuddles and general intimacy. I get up for morning walk and tasks. He still sleeps. I return to bed mid-morning for reading the paper and more cuddling. We move into more sexual activity. Sufficient erection for penetration and orgasm on his part.

Sunday

Usual wake up call. It happens quite well. No orgasm for me. Not worried—enjoyable all the same. Back to sleep until 7. Before the operation, we had sex about ten times a week. We are back on deck a year down the track—about six times weekly. I doubt if we will ever get back to pre-operation capacity. But I'm not complaining.

Monday

Early waking, usual routine sex. A bit difficult to determine who initiates. When we are both sufficiently awake—a bit of both, but usually him. Kissing, cuddling, stroking, usual scissors position. He has orgasm, but because of operation is dry orgasm. Cuddle and back to sleep for about an hour or so.

Tuesday

As for Monday. Home during day by myself. After lunch nap. Self-stimulation—decent orgasm. I needed it. Why did I take so long to really enjoy this?

Wednesday

As for Monday/Tuesday. If this seems routine or boring, we are quite happy. This is what happens 95 per cent of the time. Most of our sex is routine, everyday sex. More advanced stuff for when we are relaxed, on holiday etc. Over the years we have had episodes of very intense sex, then go back to everyday sex. We have made sure we have set aside time for sex. Have had sex for cure for insomnia, tension release and when he was depressed. Didn't know how else I could help him through that time. That is in the past I hope. Recreational sex—we have had good times, knowing that the more sex in a marriage the better.

They are doing just fine. But we have to remember that Meg is hardly a typical fifty-six year old. She belongs to that rare group of older women who remain juicy tomatoes, who don't experience the drop-off in sexual drive typical of most women, particularly those in her post-menopausal age group. And she loves bonking. That meant she was holding her breath while waiting for her husband's delicious, firm erections and strong sex drive to make a comeback.

However, there are many, many women who would welcome the penis being put out to pasture—women who have lost interest in sex; women who prefer Irma Kurtz's loving, languorous way of sex where the strutting, thrusting penis is an unwelcome intruder; women who believe that only the young should be interested in sex.[6] 'Sex—that's all you ever think of. Start acting your age!' 65-year-old Molly told her husband, 66-year-old Wayne.

There's a very good reason why many women greet the idea of Viagra with a shudder. A new lease of their sex life is the very last thing they want. Remember Nick, the 53-year-old retired police officer from Chapter 1 who held back tears of frustration over his non-existent sex life? He hasn't had sex for nearly five years. His wife is only forty-eight but has no sex drive, and he's having problems getting and maintaining an erection: 'I'm an epileptic and take Tegretol twice a day. I believe this medication is causing my erectile problems. Because I can't get an erection we do not attempt sex'. He's talking about intercourse—he does still sometimes make love to his wife. 'I perform oral sex on my wife and she tells me that's all she needs. She has the best orgasm still', he says. He has a script for Cialis and would love to try it but is stymied by his wife's indifference.

It's a common problem, says Dr Rosie King, who has helped many couples learn to adjust to this complex interaction of personal wants and needs. Ever since Viagra and the newer impotence drugs were introduced, therapists have had to deal with women who greet the prospect of a rejuvenated sex life with dread. Men who start taking the impotence drugs often find themselves confronting significant resistance from partners who were relieved that sex was no longer on the agenda. 'Some women ask the GP to take their husbands off the medication; others feel intensely guilty for not wanting sex', says King, reporting that partners' reservations have proven a major factor in men giving up on the drugs.[7]

Women often don't understand how shattered the man might feel because of his sexual failure. If he has retreated from the relationship as a result of the blow to his self-esteem, this often undermines the couple's closeness and intimacy. According to King:

> It can be shocking for a woman who has been living in a sexless relationship for years to be confronted with a full-on erection again. Instead of enthusiasm for a renewed sex life, an older woman who has got used to her personal space and a companionate relationship is likely to greet this troublesome renewed erection with a cold spoon. Other women fear that their husband, rather than wanting to make love to her again, simply wants to jump in the sack and prove his new-found masculinity.[8]

The key to resolving these problems is honesty and communication, explains King:

> Couples need to talk and be open. Women need to understand why it is so important to men to maintain that sexual connection and explore ways of revitalising their own interest. But men must tread gently not to ride rough-shod over the woman's needs and feelings. You need to work hard to rebuild trust and intimacy.[9]

King adds that now that we have drugs which offer men a second chance for having firm erections, it's natural that most men will find that opportunity irresistible.

Most—but not all. Among my diarists was a man who very happily took the other path and is living a very fulfilling sex life without an erection in sight.

David and Margaret are the Melbourne couple from Chapter 11 who were rather surprised when David's urologist asked Margaret whether she liked being poked. This was just prior to David's prostate surgery, and the doctor was trying to find out how the couple would cope if he became impotent as a result. That's precisely what happened and, as it turns out, it hasn't proven much of a problem. Penetration was never a big deal for Margaret:

> Intercourse had never been my favourite part of sex. I don't think I have ever had an orgasm that way. I have mine through digital work on the clitoris, with the help of my fantasies. Not only does intercourse NOT turn me on, but it's hard for D to rub me, I feel pinioned when he's on top of me and I don't have any room to manoeuvre. I know I used to have to work pretty hard to get any pleasure from D being in me. The right parts of my anatomy weren't getting the stimulation. God knows, he tried!

Margaret was, however, relieved to discover that David would still be able to climax:

> My concern was that if D could not ejaculate, how would we bring a sexual interaction to a close? I knew that ejaculations were the point at which I could anticipate a cuddle and a sleep. I was very much surprised and relieved to hear that D could have an orgasm without ejaculating. Wow! Not only would I get to sleep, but there would be no mess afterwards. Bonus.

Margaret's reaction is most likely far from unusual. What was more surprising was David's relaxed attitude to the prospect of life without erections:

I didn't think I needed an erection to feel good about myself. I have always felt OK about myself as a man. Nor have I lost any of my appreciation of the female form, my libido, my constant desire for Margaret. The only losses are the internal feedback I think I got from an erection when aroused and the inability to penetrate. Apart from that I'm the same guy as the pre-op guy.

David confirms that the couple's sexual life actually seems to have improved since the operation:

Now, without penetration our sexual life feels much the same. I touch Margaret in much the same way and she seems to get the same if not more pleasure. Whereas I would have generally had an orgasm during penetration, now we use a variety of manual stimulation together for me to achieve orgasm. I feel very satisfied with this and Margaret seems happy to provide help. I think she actually feels less pressure—perhaps literally —now that she doesn't have an erect penis pushing against her at night. However, she has not become less responsive. In fact, she seems more responsive and freer than ever!

Margaret's more relaxed attitude has led to quite a different relationship with David's penis:

I now welcome feeling his penis softly fitting wherever it happens to settle. In the past such a position would have instigated the swelling to a hard insistent block. I'd feel the need to respond to its wants or alternatively to feel harsh and somewhat guilty about ignoring it by turning over or falling asleep.

So here's a woman who finds it much easier to live with a penis that is soft and vulnerable rather than one that is hard and demanding—and, luckily, her partner is happy to keep it that way.

I am reminded of an interesting exercise developed by the late Bernie Zilbergeld, a well-known San Francisco sex therapist. Zilbergeld was trying to teach men who were experiencing erectile problems to tune in to their feelings. He devised a therapy exercise that required men to imagine what it would be like to be their penis, and then write a letter from their penis to themselves, the penis owner. The specific questions the man had to answer were 'How does my owner mistreat me?' and 'How could my owner treat me better?' Here's a letter Zilbergeld received from one man, or, should I say, from the penis of one of the men:

> I'm sick and tired of being called names and threatened. Don't you think I have feelings? I try to do my best and you don't do a damn thing for me or yourself. You get me into the weirdest sexual situations anyone can imagine and expect me to perform. And when I refuse, you get all huffy and start yelling at me. Christ, you don't even like most of the women you want me to screw! And do you ever ask how I feel about them? Never! Well, to hell with you, Charlie. I'm putting you on notice right now. Either you start treating me with some respect and get into situations that interest both of us, or I'm never going to do anything for you again.[10]

It's pretty funny stuff, but Zilbergeld uses the letters to help men understand what their penises are trying to tell them:

> If your penis doesn't work the way you want it to, remember it's trying to tell you something. It's not your enemy. It was made for sex, it likes sex. If it's not working the way you like, it's telling you that there is something wrong with the way you are going about sex. If you want better sex, you need to start deciphering your penis' message.[11]

Zilbergeld was onto something. Even though we now know that many men's erectile problems are due to bodily malfunctions rather than just their heads, the psyche is still hugely important. It often comes as a huge shock to a man when his erections fall prey to his emotions—anxiety, fear and indifference are all very effective passion-killers.

It strikes me that it is often difficult for women to understand the intense and complex relationship between a man and his penis. It starts as a love affair—just watch little boys who can't keep their hands from clutching their pants. But then men gradually learn that the penis has a mind, a will of its own. As teenagers, they find that it leaps into life at the most inappropriate moments, before hitting its stride as the source of a young man's greatest pleasure. But man's misfortune is that his penis, that proud and strutting proof of his sexual power, is also one of the most fragile and vulnerable organs of his body. His weapon is also his weak spot, as he soon learns when it starts to betray him.

This is all so different from women's experience of their sexuality. We don't have to live with this very public indicator of our sexual interest. For males, the penis is always there, ready to reveal their true feelings to the world and to themselves.

There's a wonderful essay by Julius Lester called 'Being a Boy', which talks about the catastrophe which befalls him when he touches the hand of a girl he has asked to dance—he has an instant, very obvious erection:

> God, how I envied girls at that moment. Whatever it was on them, it didn't dangle between their legs like an elephant's trunk. No wonder men talked about nothing but sex. That thing was always there. Every time we went to the john, there *it* was, twitching around like a little fat worm on a fishing hook. When we took baths, it floated in the water like a lazy fish and God forbid we should touch it! It sprang to life like lightning leaping from a cloud. I wished I could cut it off, or at least keep it tucked between my legs as if it were a tail that was mistakenly attached to the wrong end. But I was helpless. It was there, with a life and mind of its own, having no other function than to embarrass me.[12]

'Having no other function than to embarrass me.' And the older men get, the more likely it is that the penis will do just that. For the one in two men who hit fifty and find that their penis starts letting them down, the result can be more than embarrassment. The ensuing sense of loss, anxiety and depression can be intense and soul-destroying.

Is it any wonder that men, having spent their lives with such a capricious penis, delight in the new drugs that miraculously bring it under control? 'Now man can hold his manhood in his hand, confident in knowing who is in charge', wrote David Friedman in his cultural history of the penis, *A Mind of Its Own*. Friedman, despite some qualms, defends the medicalised penis as a giant leap forward for mankind. To argue that older men don't need rock-hard erections—a line taken by many therapists—is to deny human nature, suggests Friedman: 'if not human nature, then male nature'.[13]

We live at a sad moment in history when so many older men with a new sexual lease of life are brought swiftly to earth by sexually disinterested partners. Even if a magic bullet arrived to answer some women's prayers, rest assured there'll be plenty of others who will still prefer to close up shop.

14

Bad Health, Thinking It Is Silly and No Bicycle

Weird counting rituals. Washing hands repeatedly. These days everyone has heard of obsessive-compulsive disorders. Remember Jack Nicholson as the misanthropic novelist in *As Good as It Gets*, whose life was controlled by his compulsions, turning the lock on his door five times, avoiding cracks and lines on sidewalks and floors, throwing away gloves and bars of soap after one use?

But how about having sex only on Sunday mornings at 9.15 a.m.? That's a new one. When 68-year-old Tony from Albury first wrote to me, he warned that he couldn't promise much of a diary: Sunday 9.15 a.m., that's it. 'That's our sex diary', he told me. 'And you can ink it in for most Sundays!'

His wife, Ruth, has anxiety problems which came to a head with a major breakdown a few years ago. Tony says: 'We never want to go through anything like that ever again. Ruth was not able to do anything without help, couldn't eat properly and lost so much weight that I really feared for her ongoing health'. Sex was just not on the agenda, he tells me. But then he adds:

> No, that's not right. Ruth would cuddle up to me in bed and ask me to do it, 'because you need to'. Bit hard to perform under those circumstances. I like to think that I contribute my share to our partnership but I have never felt quite so helpless and am still learning how to deal with it. My poor girl slowly

got better and we started to make love again, rather than doing it just to satisfy a need. I still had to be very careful how and when I approached the subject but we were getting there.

Tony explains that Ruth still struggles with some obsessive-compulsive behaviour:

> One of the downsides of this rotten disease is that now every-thing has to be to a rigid routine. We are gradually overcoming this too, in many aspects of day to day life, but sex has become a once a week thing. After breakfast every Sunday morning is her allocated time—she has always preferred sex in the mornings. This is OK up to a point but I sometimes find it very hard to stop whatever I am doing and go back to bed! It's fine once we get going but a bit more spontaneity would be great. Word of this seems to have got around the family and they all know not to ring up Sunday mornings.

This is a couple who have been through the mill—Ruth has a history of illness stretching back through seven operations for ovarian cysts, a hysterectomy and a major back operation, even before the anxiety issue took hold. Tony says they ran into problems with sex early in their 41-year marriage:

> I can still vividly recall my wife sitting in bed crying tears of frustration which used to tear me apart but I was still equally frustrated not knowing what to do. We tried doctors, and anyone we thought may be able to help … Useless! Ruth wondered if she was getting 'frigid', a term much used in those days. Finally we saw a friend who was a specialist in Melbourne. He gave her a course of injections to pick up her libido. It did increase her desire, but not for me!!
>
> That was a bit of a shock but it ran its course, the third party left the district and wounds started to heal. Like all these things, it was not one-sided and I think that I was a lot to blame. When my needs were not met I got very resentful. However, one good

kick in the backside did wonders for my concentration on my family and we muddled on.

Then came the breakthrough. It was my own sex magazine, *Forum*, which ultimately brought an end to Ruth's frustration, Tony tells me—'We discovered *Forum* and I was able to bring my wife to orgasm for the first time after almost ten years together'.

Despite everything, the couple still has a great sex life—every Sunday at 9.15 a.m.:

> Once we get going it's great!! Ruth enjoys an orgasm most of the time and while I struggle a bit with the regularity of it, for a couple of oldies, it works. We are an affectionate couple with plenty of cuddles but no amount of that will lead to anything on any other day.

Tony's story has added a little something to my own Sunday mornings. If I happen to notice a clock around that time, I always think of that Albury couple and smile. It is inspiring that despite all of their health issues, sex remains a comfort, a means of connection, which they both value.

'The things that stop you enjoying sex in old age are the same things that stop you riding a bicycle: bad health, thinking it is silly and no bicycle.' These words of wisdom come from Alex Comfort's 1972 bestseller, *The Joy of Sex*.[1] Comfort gets it pretty right. While we are getting over our hang-ups about sex in old age, bad health can derail even the most active and enjoyable of love lives. My diarists bear witness to that. Ruth's anxiety problem is only one of a long list of health issues that play havoc with desire, with mental health problems like depression now ranking as the most serious.

Melbourne man Matthew (aged fifty-six) has good reason to be depressed. Five years ago, he had an accident requiring a series of operations to repair a nearly severed foot. Since then life has been rather a struggle, which has taken its toll on his libido:

Since recovering, I have gone from having a normal sex drive to it being practically non-existent. This worries me as far as being a normal sexual partner for my wife. We have discussed this and even though she says it's OK, I think she would prefer otherwise. We have gone from three times per month to once every three or four months, and even then it is a 'quickie'.

Matthew and Jane have been married for thirty-four years and despite what's happened, they still have a lot of fun together. They get on extremely well and very much enjoy each other's company. 'We are lucky in that we have a really close relationship together, no hang-ups about being naked in front of the other; we shower together, massage each other and touch each other throughout the night in bed: everything is there except the physical act of making love', says Matthew.

Matthew has been diagnosed with clinical depression and is on medication, which he feels isn't helping very much: 'I can't seem to shake the black dog off. He is becoming a constant companion of late. And sex is just not on the radar; I would rather watch TV or read in bed'. He assures me that this has nothing to do with Jane, but rather a whole host of other things: 'a state of mind that I can't explain, maybe pain, medication, lack of physical exercise, a hard time in our lives being incapacitated and with Jane being the carer as well as working'.

Matthew says that they don't find it easy to discuss the decline in his drive: 'Jane and I have talked about this and she says it's not an issue. I have found that discussing our sex life is quite difficult: the blame thing creeps in and one of us gets the huffs and that's the end of it. The issue is left standing'.

Then there's Harriet (aged twenty-five), who is about to get married. Her man has depression. 'He's on antidepressants and smokes and drinks and has no libido whatsoever', she says. Four weeks from their wedding day, they are having sex less than once a month.

Elisa (aged twenty-eight) has been married for five years. She's been through periods when she had a very high drive—'I've had about twenty-five partners', she reports. When she first met Owen, she was the one who wanted sex more. But now that's all changed. 'I suffer from depression and my medication has caused my libido to go AWOL. Combine that with having kids and poor Owen has been copping the short end of the stick', she writes cheerfully.

Helen is in her early sixties, married for the third time. She writes:

> My desire for sex has diminished for the past two years and it is now at almost zero level. I have recently commenced medication for depression to try to assist my moods and thus my desire, but am now discovering that medication may have some effect on lowering my libido! That's depressing!

According to beyondblue, a government-supported mental health organisation, depression now affects one in five Australians, so it is hardly surprising to find it emerging as the number one health issue reported by my diarists.[2] They see a strong link between depression and loss of desire, a connection now backed up by strong research evidence. Yet the exact mechanism whereby depression impacts on sex drive has yet to be determined. In fact, treatment for depression may be causing more problems than the disease, at least when we are looking at people's sex lives. Some of the major antidepressant drugs—particularly the SSRIs (selective serotonin reuptake inhibitors)—are known to all but abolish desire in some patients. Some studies indicate that as many as 50 per cent of people on SSRIs suffer a markedly reduced sex drive.

Researchers believe that SSRIs quash libido by flooding the bloodstream with serotonin, a chemical that signals satiety. The drugs also place a dampener on the libido-enhancing effects of falling in love, according to anthropologist Helen Fisher. Fisher's research suggests that when SSRIs elevate the level of serotonin in the synapses of the brain, they suppress the dopamine circuits that are activated when people fall for each other. The dopamine circuits are central to the elation, the obsessive thinking associated with the limerence stage of romantic love. Fisher argues that SSRIs blunt those emotions, interfering with natural courtship—one study found that women taking SSRIs rated male faces as less attractive than women not using the drugs, a process known as 'courtship blunting'.[3]

The good news is that there are antidepressants that act through other channels. NDRIs (norepinephrine dopamine reuptake inhibitors) boost two neurotransmitters, and early research suggests they may actually enhance libido in women. There are also drugs known as SSNRIs (selective serotonin norepinephrine reuptake inhibitors) which add norepinephrine to the mix, resulting in less negative effects on libido. So there are alternative drugs available if depression medication seems to be reducing sex drive.

But antidepressants are only the beginning of the story. There's a long, long list of other medication that can also play havoc with libido:

o some blood pressure medications

o tranquillisers

o benzodiazepines

o steroids

o some diuretics

o some anti-ulcer medications

o beta-blockers

o antipsychotics

o appetite suppressors

o some antihistamines.

The contraceptive pill is another culprit, though not for all women. Many of my diarists who took the high-dose Pill twenty to thirty years ago report that this interfered with their drive. But even a slight increase in the hormone level can be enough to disrupt libido for some women.

Adrianne (aged forty) wrote to me reporting that she had had over twenty years of putting up with the creeping hand, checking out if she was in the mood for love. 'Ugh. It still sends a shiver down my spine', she writes. But then she made her move. 'I left my marriage aged thirty-eight. I was sure that sex could be nice and could last longer than a couple of minutes. Those Hollywood movies couldn't all be wrong? Surely?', says Adrianne. She struck it lucky: 'I met the man of my dreams, and he has patiently coached me and encouraged me and now I LOVE SEX. I love the intimacy. I love the pure pleasure. He loves sex. I love sex. It's all good. (I even get turned down sometimes)'.

The one time she experienced a glitch in her current relationship was when she changed her brand of Pill:

> Interestingly enough, I was not really interested in sex for a three-month period (we've been together for two-and-a-half years) and couldn't even get 'ready'. I had been on the 20 milligram birth control pill, tried the 30 milligram as it was cheaper, and then when we realised the side effects of low libido and nausea, went straight back to the 20 milligram—and back to how our sex life was before.

Of course, there are other issues relating to reproduction which can also interfere with desire—like unwanted pregnancy. Anthea (aged thirty-three) from Melbourne is one of my juicy tomatoes, a woman who describes herself as having a 'stupidly high sex drive'. Since leaving her marriage three years ago, she has revelled in her new-found, intense sexual interest, as her raunchy early diaries showed. But then came a very different letter:

I am not sure if this is appropriate for your research but it has greatly impacted upon my sexuality, my desire for sex and my relationship with my partner so I am going to share it with you. I have not had sex or even masturbated for close to two weeks now, which is incomprehensible for me. The reason behind this is because, even though I have done a pregnancy test and it was negative, I fear I am pregnant. I have always practised safe sex but about three weeks ago the condom broke and now I am in that horrible limbo of not being sure.

It turned out she was indeed pregnant—the very last thing she wanted:

I am so angry, in every respect. I looked at pregnancy tests and they all showed happy smiling women. Why are women supposed to be happy when they are pregnant? Is that all we are seen to be here for? The thought of losing my body to a pregnancy fills me with fear and dread. I feel partly selfish but I feel I will lose myself as a sexual being. I once asked a GP to allow me to go for a tubal ligation but they said I was too young. Typical male arrogance. The stress of thinking I may be pregnant has completely taken any sexual urge whatsoever from me.

Anthea has two children from a previous relationship and has no desire for any more:

I am so angered with my partner that I have planned to meet with one of my lovers. It is partly because of the way he has reacted to the situation. His small smile when I told him was almost one of triumph. He had not been able to have any control over the relationship and now with the possibility of him having impregnated me due to a faulty condom, I am suddenly at his mercy. I will not have it!

Anthea ended up having a termination.

At the other extreme were the couples struggling to fall pregnant—I had half a dozen in this situation. And despite the fact that this meant that most were having plenty of sex, generally they reported that it didn't do much for their sex drive. 'We have gone through stages where sex is the last thing we want to do', writes Amanda (aged thirty), also from Melbourne. She and Kevin have been trying to conceive for the past year—they both have children from previous relationships but were keen to have a child together—and it is taking its toll on their great sex life.

Ten months after they first started writing for me, they both report they are still very happy, but the strain is showing. Here's Kevin, reporting how trying to make a baby is having a 'strange' effect on their lovemaking:

> Even though it should be a loving time, I find it places an enormous amount of pressure on me. Even though I am only half of the equation, I feel that we haven't been able to conceive yet due to something being not quite right with me. A couple of months ago, I went and had my swimmers tested. We had already been to see a fertility specialist, and we knew that Amanda was ovulating, and to be honest, I don't think the problem is with her. I think that the biggest thing for me was the fact that I used to smoke. I know that that is going to affect sperm count and motility, so when my test results came back a little lower than normal, I wasn't all that surprised. The doctor I spoke to on the phone did say that I was basically in the normal range, and that we should just go and do IVF. She was very abrupt, and really pissed me off with her demeanour, so at that point, I pretty much decided that I was over it.
>
> When we were having sex around the time of ovulation, I would find that my mind would not always be on the fact that we were making love. Instead I was wondering whether this month would work, whereas others had failed. It does your

head in, I can assure you, and certainly doesn't make having sex the mind-blowing experience it usually is with the woman I love.

So for the time being, they have decided to give up on all the charts and plotting cycles and just try to go with the flow, as Amanda explains:

> If I am really honest I would say that this month has really been the first month where I think we both have accepted that there may not ever be a baby. In some ways it has meant we have just enjoyed each other that much more and have made love more. Sounds ridiculous, but we have tried to plan too much, making sex every second day so that the sperm supply has time to replenish. We have thrown everything out this month and are in a better place for it.

So our efforts to control reproduction are a major part of the libido story. But there is also a long list of physical conditions that are known to affect sexual drive, including fatigue, physical tension, acute and chronic pain, chronic heart or lung disease, acute or chronic infection, auto-immune disease, recurrent urinary tract and vaginal infections, kidney, thyroid and liver disease, cancer, blood disorders, metabolic disease, hormone disturbance and chromosomal abnormalities. You can add to these the known sexual hazards of indulging in too much alcohol, smoking, taking various illicit drugs and becoming severely overweight.

Oh yes, there are plenty of good health-related reasons for going off sex, and they featured strongly in the diaries. Dan (aged forty-two) says: 'I tried the cuddling thing again. Susan complained of a back pain and that was that'. Antonia (aged fifty-eight) reports: 'As my husband began to drink more he didn't care if I wanted sex or not. I was turned off sex and refused to have sex at night as he had usually been drinking'.

Arthur, who is aged fifty-six, has his own health-related problems:

> My back is slowly getting better. I think my wife could be a bit more physically affectionate with stroking and gentle massage but she says, 'I can't do anything for you. I will only make it worse'. She has not touched me for more than a week. When I reach out she either moves away or does not respond at all.

She doesn't feel like it; he's too sick to do it; their bodies are breaking down and they don't feel like having sex—so it is assumed that nothing will happen. There's rarely any suggestion that they will still make the effort to give pleasure to their partners, even if they are not in the mood themselves. The whole notion of mercy sex, comfort sex, of finding some way of giving pleasure to ensure that your partner feels desired and desirable, appears to have gone out of fashion. Many people seem to have given up on the idea of making love just to show they care, and many women rankle at the thought that their partners might expect this of them.

But perhaps we need to rethink this issue. Over the years I have watched so many women friends with health problems who still cope when they have to, when they are tackling something they really want to do. Her back is killing her and she couldn't possibly make love, yet somehow she manages to stagger around the house and cook her children's dinner. Despite that dreadful arthritis, another woman is able to pick up her son from rugby practice and help him work on his science project. Even with her heart condition, a third still rushes around and cleans up the house when her mother-in-law pays a visit. Bad health does impose limitations, but we find a way around these when it really matters. How come lovemaking isn't a similar priority?

Men are just the same. A man's depression may not be enough to stop him cleaning his new car or spending hours comparison-shopping for the latest techno boy toy, but he simply doesn't have the energy to spend ten, twenty minutes lying down caressing his wife. Does this really make sense?

Luckily, there are exceptions—amazing couples who are snowed under by medical problems yet still make their sex lives a priority. These diarists brought home to me the good sense in Michele Weiner Davis's argument that desire is a decision. As the body starts to deteriorate, it is very easy to come up with good reasons why we are not interested in sex. Weiner Davis points out that there are plenty of people who are experts on why they have been avoiding sexual contact with their spouse. Yet, as she says, knowing why you are not interested in sex won't boost your desire one bit; doing something about it will.[4]

One extraordinary couple, Jim and Amy from Brisbane, are certainly proof of that. It was Jim who greeted me at the door of their well-kept suburban house and ushered me into the living room, where Amy was seated, both her legs in plaster. She has a form of rheumatoid arthritis, peripheral neuropathy and a condition that causes the bones of her feet to disintegrate. The result is that she is in constant pain—this varies from 'bearable to excruciating', she says. Amy (aged fifty-four) is the woman introduced in Chapter 5 who spent her early marriage dreading the hand creeping across the bed, seeking sex. The couple spent the first ten years of their marriage fighting about sex—he always wanted it, she never did. If she refused him, she'd suffer the consequences: 'I'd lie awake at night thinking, "I might as well have let him have it". He would take it out on me somehow, by not talking to me, showing me I was in the bad books'. 'She said she could always tell by the curl of my lip whether I was angry or happy', Jim (aged fifty-six) says with a rueful laugh.

It became a dreadful problem but they never talked about it. Then their lives were struck by a major disaster—they lost a child, a little boy born with a heart defect. The death came after many months of enormous strain. 'We had to be with him twenty-four hours a day. One of us would sleep four hours and get up and the other would sleep. Then he died. Those years are a bit of a blur. I can't really remember what our sex life was like', says Amy.

Six months after their son died they were still in the depths of grief, hardly talking to one another. 'I didn't want to say anything because it would upset Jim and he didn't want to say anything because it would upset me. I had lost a son and nearly lost my husband because we literally weren't talking', remembers Amy. But then a friend suggested they attend a marriage encounter weekend designed to help couples communicate. Amy says:

> We did the weekend and it just saved our lives. It was as if we had started again, started from scratch. It took our marriage to a level we hadn't been before. We cried from the moment we walked in the door to the moment we left, we had so much grief bottled up. How they put up with us I don't know.

Amy chuckles but it is very clear it was a huge relief that they found each other again. And they also rediscovered their sex life. Amy explains that they started to talk about what was going on between them:

> Instead of waiting until we got to bed and the hand reaching over, he would say, 'How about it?' That gave me the opportunity to say, 'I would love to but I have to get up in the morning early tomorrow', to tell him what I was feeling rather than nothing being spoken and just refusing with him having no idea what was going on.

As they talked about it, Amy had a brainwave. She came up with the idea of scheduling sex: 'I sat Jim down and said, "How long can you go without sex without climbing up the wall?"' Four days, was his answer. Amy knew she couldn't cope with sex every night so they compromised by settling on every third night. 'I got out the diary and put a red S every three days', says Amy. That was to be the arrangement while they were still in their thirties—they decided they would drop that back to every fourth day when they were in their forties, every fifth day in their fifties and so on. 'I thought, "Wow, that means I'll still be getting it once a week in my seventies"', Jim chips in.

It worked wonderfully for them. 'It was so freeing for both of us. From my perspective I knew every three days there would be this wonderful occasion. I knew I could give Amy a cuddle on the other two days and know she appreciated it, know there was no point getting excited', Jim explains. Amy adds:

> Jim is a very affectionate, touchy-feely person but he tended to push himself away because he knew I would think any cuddle meant sex was inevitable. Once sex was in the diary he became incredibly affectionate. I'd have three days to work myself up to the S Day, to ensure that everything about the day was just right. I'd ring him up from work … nudge, nudge, wink, wink. Tonight's the night. We both found it incredibly liberating.

The other big breakthrough involved a change in Amy's thinking. As she explained in Chapter 5, she suddenly realised she didn't need desire to enjoy sex. Once Amy got over the stumbling block of thinking that she had to want it first, she found she could enjoy sex and all would be fine.

The couple's sex life then flourished until Amy's recent health problems. It was very sad hearing how her painful condition has interfered with their regular lovemaking. About a year before they first wrote to me, Jim moved out of the shared bed into another room, so that Amy could be more comfortable during her difficult nights—but strictly on the understanding that he still had 'visiting rights'. Amy says she has tried to keep up their schedule but recently has often had to renege because of severe back pain. It has become almost impossible for her to participate in intercourse, so they have had to be satisfied with mutual masturbation—'Even that can be too difficult for me if my back is particularly bad', she says. That's a loss for Amy, who has always enjoyed vaginal orgasm:

> If I am pain-free, after experiencing a clitoral orgasm I feel what I've read described as a 'hungry vagina' and can then experience a vaginal orgasm (or several). All our married life, J has been totally considerate and waited for me to give the cue for intercourse. I'm sure that's why we have had such a great sex life.

It is touching reading their diaries, as they express their constant concern for each other while struggling to maintain regular physical intimacy. It is so obvious that they still lust after each other—they sit close together on the couch as I talk with them, touching, laughing, so clearly closely connected despite their current difficulties. 'I can look at my wonderful wife, or even think about her, at any time of the day or night, and have wonderful thoughts of wonderful things with her', writes Jim, explaining that he goes to the gym several mornings a week and tackles 'bushwalking like a mad thing—all designed to try to lessen my sexual desire'.

Amy wants so much to be able to make love with him, but is naturally fearful of the consequences for her health.

Tuesday, 17 April 2007—Amy's diary

I was still pain-free and thinking that I could take the opportunity to have sex tonight. Whenever J and I were together, I was unusually affectionate (kissing, stroking etc.). I was feeling amorous and wanting to convey the message to J that I was thinking about sex. However, I was still in two minds whether to issue an invitation to J or enjoy another painless night's sleep. I did eventually decide to risk some lovemaking; even though

I was frightened it would set my back off again. When the time came, I decided to forget my fears and go for broke. We had a fantastic time and my back was still OK in the morning!

Sunday, 22 April 2007

Even though my back was beginning to get sore again, I was thinking that it would be a good idea to try to get back to a reasonable 'schedule' while we had the opportunity. We had had a lovely weekend celebrating friends' birthdays and J had been very loving and attentive towards me. I invited him into my bed for some lovemaking, but he turned me down, saying that I needed to take care of my back. I said I was willing to give it a try, but he still refused. I was in a quandary—wanting to give J some pleasure, but also nervous about my back. I don't want my health to jeopardise our relationship.

Thursday, 26 April 2007

Pain getting unbearable again and we're due to go away for the weekend. I called in at physio to see if I could get some more electrical treatment and they did it for me on the spot—instant relief! I can now look forward to the weekend, except for having to sleep in a strange bed. No question of any sex tonight, as I have to ensure that my back is as good as possible for the weekend.

Sunday, 29 April 2007

Home from the weekend away and I knew I simply had to invite J into my bed—it's been nearly two weeks and he must be desperate! What bliss to be back in my own bed. I tried to fully participate in our lovemaking but found I just couldn't. Perhaps I was too tired after the drive home, or perhaps the nerve damage caused by my spinal condition has reached the genital area. At least J had some relief and I was able to sleep well.

Jim writes to me a few weeks later, expressing his concern about what's happening:

> I really thought Sunday 6 May was going to be 'the last', as Amy said after our lovemaking that 'she doesn't feel much down there any more'. So last Sunday, when Amy made the offer, I refused. Because of her health, we sleep in separate beds (that was a grief process for me when it first happened), so the offer always comes from her: 'Do you want to sleep in my bed tonight?'
>
> Our routine for the last couple of years consists of mutual stimulation to orgasm. Only occasionally do we enjoy penetrative sex and after every time, Amy suffers pretty badly. Over the last few months she hasn't even been able to orgasm, so I have the feeling that she's doing it just for me, even though she says she enjoys the cuddle. I have feelings of guilt (because my barely diminished libido is causing Amy to offer lovemaking); grief (because what we have enjoyed for so many years is passing); yet confidence that we can adjust to a new routine that will see us forward.

There was no correspondence for a while, until Amy finally reported that her health had declined still further:

> Since I last wrote my back has deteriorated significantly. I have severe arthropathy of the lumbar spine, to the extent that major nerves to the legs are being pinched and there is bony protrusion into the spinal canal. That means major pain! It usually takes about two hours in the morning before my legs will work and by evening they give up again. Lying in bed is hell, so I have to drug myself to the eyeballs to manage a few hours of broken sleep. Needless to say, our sex life isn't crash hot!

Amy says that Jim is extremely understanding:

> He never puts any demand or expectation on me. He knows that, if and when I can, I will instigate our lovemaking. While

we were away, strange beds made everything even worse for me, so, most of the time, I couldn't get involved enough to achieve orgasm, but I was happy for him to have some release. Now that we're home, I've worked out that I can medicate myself sufficiently to relieve the pain and, as long as we're reasonably quick, we can both have a good time before I fall asleep!

So here she is, hardly able to walk and in constant pain, yet still she is determined to try to maintain a regular sex life:

I am still trying to maintain a regularity of once a week, unless it is absolutely impossible. Why? Well, it's certainly not because of any fear that J would be unfaithful. There is an element of wanting to keep him happy—I am very aware that, after about a week, he seems to become more and more distant, even grumpy. But I think the main motivation is that I believe that sex is an essential part of marriage—it maintains a sense of intimacy between us which permeates everything we do. I feel that, without sex, we would simply be two people living under the same roof, and I don't want that to happen to our marriage.

Both Amy and Jim are religious people and work in their church, offering sex and marriage counselling. During counselling they talk about their own experiences, to help young couples learn how to work through the problems they might encounter in their marriages. What an inspiration they must be. I often think about this couple—remembering their ease with each other, their sexy banter and their determination to not allow Amy's battle with her deteriorating body to drive them apart. It makes all of our usual excuses, like the classic 'Not tonight dear, I've got a headache', seem very lame indeed.

15

The Desire to Desire

It was the *Annie Hall* movie that triggered the idea. Friends were chatting about that very funny scene mentioned in Chapter 1, where Woody Allen and Diane Keaton discuss with their therapists their contrasting views on sexual frequency. I had an inspiration—why not ask couples to write diaries about their negotiations over the sex supply, to find out what really was going on in bedrooms around the country? The rest came easily. People flocked to volunteer after I went on radio and wrote a magazine article seeking out people who would write for me. I talked about the sexually deprived men who craved more sex, the uninterested women who dreaded that creeping hand crossing the bed. So many of the hundreds of couples who made contact with me were just delighted to discover that someone knew what they were going through. 'I have passed the link to my husband today with the words "Hooray, I'm not the only one!"' wrote one woman.

As the words started to pour in, I realised I was onto something big. The sex supply proved to be a huge issue for so many couples, a gaping wound in the goodwill and intimacy of their relationships. Even for couples who were normally harmonious, people who enjoyed the company of their partners, sex could become a constant, unvoiced source of tension. The men were the real surprise. Their diaries revealed their misery and bewilderment over the fact that their most basic desire—to share physical intimacy with their loved one—so often was being ignored or treated with disdain. And most women knew it. While many expressed irritation at their partner's relentless sexual drive, many felt guilty about the pattern of rejection in their nightly encounters. Handling the discrepancies in sexual desire turned out to be one of the major battlegrounds in marriage today.

Ninety-eight couples were keen to tell me all about it. It was an amazing experience, spending a year peering into Australia's bedrooms. I could hardly wait to get to my computer each day, to study the latest batch of emailed diaries. I ended up getting to know some people very well as they emailed day after day, with occasional phone calls when they hit bumpy patches. Sometimes I couldn't resist an actual meeting, as with the hot young Sydney woman who'd written pages and pages about her lover, as she struggled to persuade her husband to be attentive. I had coffee with Sally from Queensland—the 'good, safe Catholic girl gone bad'—and helped her buy new red boots on Oxford Street, just the thing for her nights out dancing in her local pub. I travelled to meet the Melbourne couple whose sex life was flourishing despite erections being off the menu, and the Adelaide pair with their twenty-three years of diaries—what a treat to be allowed to see Heather's sexy underwear drawer and to rustle through the treasure trove of satin and lace.

Some sent pages and pages of handwritten notes which arrived by snail mail. But email suited most of the diarists, who'd often crawl out of bed last thing at night to describe their most recent bout of activity. A few were writing in secret, with their partners totally unaware that their every sexual move was being documented and used for research. But most couples did it together, seeing the research as a means of learning more about their own relationship. Some couples took turns at the computer, each filing their own stories. 'We giggled like teenagers when we were doing it', reported Kevin and Amanda from Melbourne. That's not surprising. These two had plenty to smile about. They had been together less than a year when they first contacted me. Kevin, the loquacious one, wrote over seventy pages of diary entries describing in great detail their joyous sexual encounters.

How sad that this lust so rarely lasts. That was the most powerful message to emerge from the sex diaries. So many of my couples could look back to the early stage of their own history and report rutting like rabbits, not being able to keep their hands off each other. But a few years later, many ran into problems as desire discrepancies started to affect couples' mutual generosity and goodwill. That's the terrible thing—the actual lovemaking isn't the problem: it's the impact that tension over sex has on closeness and intimacy that is at the heart of the matter. It's just one of life's dirty tricks.

There's a very nice joke about Albert Einstein arriving at the Pearly Gates. The Good Lord greets him and asks whether he has any questions. 'How did you create all this? The animals, people, the whole world?' Einstein inquires. God produces a blackboard and starts writing an enormous equation, filling up the entire board. Einstein looks at it, frowns and shakes his head, saying, 'But, my Lord, there are so many mistakes'. 'You're telling me', God replies.

Are we to assume that the mismatch in desire so frequently felt in relationships is simply a design flaw? That the Good Lord stuffed up when he paired men and their strong, eternal-flame libidos with women and their damp-wood drives? Evolutional psychologists like Helen Fisher argue that it was simply meant to be. 'We are an animal that wasn't built to be happy. We were built to reproduce', she asserts cheerfully.[1] Some of her colleagues argue that women's low drive is designed to ensure they keep their eyes on the job—namely the demanding business of caring for their young—while men need constant desire to keep sowing their seeds, ensuring the survival of the species.

Dietrich Klusman has a slightly different take on the matter. He's a German evolutionary psychologist who recently studied patterns of desire and found that 60 per cent of 30-year-old women wanted sex often at the beginning of a relationship, but that within four years this figure fell to under 50 per cent, and after twenty years it dropped to about 20 per cent. In contrast, the proportion of men wanting regular sex remained between 60 to 80 per cent, regardless of how long they had been in a relationship. It's all due to human evolution, suggests Klusman:

> For men, a good reason for their sexual motivation to remain constant would be to guard against being cuckolded by another man. But women have evolved to have a high sex drive when they are initially in a relationship in order to form a 'pair bond' with their partner but once this bond is sealed a woman's sexual appetite declines.[2]

No one really knows why we have ended up this way—evolutionary psychology often simply comes down to fancy guesswork. Whatever the reason, we do seem to be left with a large divide, with strong biological differences between the sexes. Yet there are exceptions, as my juicy tomatoes and celery stick men so clearly show. We simply don't know why some women retain a burning sexual drive all their lives. Nor do we have any idea why some men have the fragile libidos normally associated with women and can lose sexual interest early in their relationships.

Then there's the 'Coolidge Effect'. That's what psychologists call men's quest for sexual variety. The name comes from a story about former US president Calvin Coolidge and his wife visiting a poultry farm. During the tour, Mrs Coolidge inquired how the farm managed to produce so many eggs with such a small number of roosters. The farmer proudly explained that his roosters performed their duty dozens of times each day. 'Perhaps you could point that out to Mr Coolidge', replied the first lady in a pointedly loud voice.

The president, overhearing the remark, asked the farmer, 'Does each rooster service the same hen each time?'

'No,' replied the farmer, 'there are many hens for each rooster'.

'Perhaps you could point that out to Mrs Coolidge', replied the president.

Sure, sexual novelty is well known for its aphrodisiacal effects on men, but we now know it works for women too. Lorraine Dennerstein's research, reported in Chapter 4, noted the boost to sexual drive that occurs when older women change partners.[3] Many of my diarists reported such a pattern, with the women who had had or were having affairs all claiming that their sexual drive remained high when rationed to infrequent sex with elusive lovers, presumably because this irregular contact ensures that the chemical fix from the 'in love' brain hormones is never given a chance to die down.

A year after she first contacted me, Rosemary from Sydney—the woman having the world's most boring affair—reports that it is still going strong:

> Eddie is the icing on my cake. I see him about once a month or so. The situation frustrates me if I allow it to but I am keenly aware of what the relationship brings to my life—excitement, a bit of adventure, the chance for a great snog. Nothing excites me more than the thought of undoing his pants, drawing out his cock and feeling him quiver as I swallow him whole. I appreciate having that to look forward to the next time we meet. Being with him makes me feel alive.

Even women who have totally lost interest in sex know that if a new man was there to tempt them, their libido might just shift back into life. Remember Mary, the woman with the dog hair–covered laundry from Chapter 9? She recently wrote to say that participating in the research has taught her to be more understanding of what makes her husband, Peter, 'tick' where sex is concerned. She picked up on the idea that 'men go to bed with their imaginations', which gave her an insight into how Peter maintains his lust for her: 'Now I understand why he can still look at me—fat, flabby, forty and coming to bed in a T-shirt, and he can still be ready for it, whereas I can't for the life of me work up any interest'. This has made her less likely to be angry at Peter when he's making a move on her, but has done nothing for her low drive. She's still 'over it':

> I feel complete with his companionship, I love his bodily warmth in bed, he truly is my heart and soul, I love him dearly and would like to grow old with him—but I live on the edge of dreading when a simple and welcome hug or gentle caress is going to turn into 'IT'. Sex has simply disappeared off my radar.

But then came a surprise postscript. 'HOLD THE PRESS!' Mary wrote:

> Recently something happened to me to make me sit up and rethink everything. I have a new boss at work and quite frankly he is absolutely edible! I'm ashamed to say I dream about him all the time. My imagination and my libido, which I'd thought was extinct, have woken up with a vengeance. In my dreams I'm leaping into bed with him and performing the sorts of sexual acts that would get me a gold in those Olympics. What is WRONG with me—why can't I get these bits of mine working for the RIGHT MAN????

That's the question that continues to haunt so many of my female diarists. They too want lust to kick in, not just when they drool over Brad Pitt or a sexy colleague at work, but for the same old partner or husband who shares their bed each night. Maybe Helen Fisher is right in suggesting that we just aren't built to stay happy in long-term relationships. But can we work at staying happy? One of the main aims of my research was to study not only the couples struggling with desire discrepancy, but also those who have learnt to deal with it. And that's been the real thrill. Biology need not be our destiny. Yes, most couples have to cope with differences in their basic levels of desire, but there are those who, despite this, still achieve sexual harmony.

Much to my surprise, the sex diary project proved mightily helpful in getting couples to that point. Many diarists reported that the act of writing down what was happening gave them new insights into their relationships and helped clarify their thinking. Ivan from near Bunbury in Western Australia writes:

> The process of putting thoughts on paper obliges you to think harder and in the process you discover other interesting aspects that were previously lurking, half-formed, in the back of your mind. Now an important area of my life is a great deal clearer. I feel grateful that I have had such a beautiful sexual relationship with my wife for thirty-odd years. Talk about counting your blessings! And my heightened awareness has increased my confidence in dealing with marital issues that could be vexatious if not handled with the utmost goodwill and care.

Many of the diarists who were at loggerheads with their partners over the sex supply when they first contacted me reported they soon began to understand each other better. 'I was never, ever aggressive towards my wife but at times I felt like exploding', writes Clive from Sydney. He goes on to say:

For many years, I had been troubled by our relationship. I loved my wife and my family. They are the cornerstone to my life. All other things are unimportant compared to them. But between my unrequited sexual needs, and her lack of sexual interest, I was going quietly insane. I started to question my state of mental health. Having an affair wasn't on the agenda. I wanted my wife. But the less I got, the more I wanted it. So what do you do? I mentally questioned why she didn't want sex. Had she fallen out of love? Was she seeing somebody else? Maybe she now wanted women rather than men. I didn't know why.

In moments when I wondered whether our relationship was over, I considered, maybe I might be better off elsewhere. That thought was often short lived, as I quickly recognised that, in fact, it was highly likely that I would end up in a similar situation, after losing a wife I loved, having a family I loved torn apart, and then ending up with somebody else and still not having my sexual/love needs met. For about two years, the anger, sadness, frustration, despair, went around and around.

It came as an immense relief to Clive to read the article I wrote when first recruiting people for my research. He discovered his sexual needs were normal, as was his wife's lack of interest.

He had great difficulty persuading his wife even to read that article: 'Eventually I basically said to her that if she still wanted a marriage she had better read it'. Clive's wife never did participate in the research but he wrote diaries, we corresponded and the couple eventually talked about what was going on between them. The tension has now eased, according to Clive:

> The fact that we were in fact pretty normal came as a relief to both of us, allowed us to get past the guilt issues and move forward with our relationship. She knows I naturally need more and I know she naturally needs less and we don't blame each other, accepting that is the way it is and looking for solutions, rather than blaming each other.

What sorts of solutions? Well, Clive explains that he always used to want his wife to orgasm first, but now he realises that isn't always the best plan:

> Now our sexual frequency has increased, and sometimes she doesn't orgasm or even want to orgasm and she allows me to make love to her, as a gift to me. Why? Because she loves me and we realise it's up to both of us to accept our differences but love our partners and find some middle ground. So now I don't feel like I'm begging for sex. She does make more of an effort and if she doesn't feel like sex, I no longer get upset, or double guess why it didn't happen. We do feel happier and more content with each other than we did twelve months ago.

Judy is the woman from Chapter 1 who complained that her sex switch was firmly in the 'off' position. She recently wrote to say she's now relieved to find that this is quite common:

> I began to see I was not some kind of freak and began to assert myself a bit more. I started to say things like, 'You know, darling, you have a very high libido and mine's always been very low, so we're not wrong, we're just different'. I believe he has gradually accepted that could be true and we have had quite a few discussions that have helped settle the angst that was always there. I don't understand why sex is just SO important to men but I have to deal with the fact that it IS and that in my marriage, part of the give and take is I give him sex when he wants it, rather than completely cut it out of our lives.

Judy adds that they are still having sex a few times a week—'Would prefer it a couple of times a month but hey, it's better than every night!'

Learning that most women experience a decline in sexual drive after the passing of that early 'in love' stage of a relationship came as a great relief to many couples, defusing the anger and confusion many had been experiencing.

Lucy and Noel were rowing constantly over sex when they first contacted me. He was extremely bitter at her denial of his needs, leading to a major rift between them. The diary process was pretty painful for this couple, as they poured their feelings out on paper. But six months after they had stopped writing, things had improved somewhat after they had finally found a way to deal with the irreconcilable differences between them. Lucy explains that:

> Noel and I are in a better place than we were when we first contacted you. After I explained to him that my loss of drive wasn't about him, but about me, then he stopped taking it so personally. He no longer nags me for sex and leaves the initiation up to me. Having said that, I still tend to initiate out of a sense of guilt rather than desire, and not nearly enough to satisfy his desires. I made a decision recently that my silently stewing over various discrepancies was only hurting me. We've dragged ourselves through the mud enough with discussions and so re-running old issues is obviously not going to make any difference either. I decided I would take the road of silent forgiveness rather than silent fury as it's far healthier. Just accepting that he is what he is and I am what I am puts us both in the position of being human and neither being at fault. I just try to forgive whatever the latest upset is and let it go, allowing me to move past it and then being able to sleep with him at night. I think we're at a place where things are OK. Not passionate or exciting, just OK. This will have to be enough for now while we're in the phase of child-rearing and bill-paying. Any developments will have to wait I guess.

It was fascinating to watch people struggle with and finally accept the limitations of their relationships, and to work through their disappointment when they found themselves confronted by ongoing tensions and disharmony. The women in particular often talked about the unrealistic expectations they had had, their yearning for a soul mate, for great sex, total intimacy and togetherness. But by the end of the research, many reported that they were able finally to stop blaming themselves or their partners and move on, enjoying what was good in the relationship.

Phoebe told me that before the diary project, she had been nervous that her marriage was doomed due to the incompatibility of her and her husband's sexual desires:

> I think having a forum within which I could be really honest about my sexual fears and desires has relieved me of some of the boogie men. I had avoided looking hard at the issues because I was scared I might come to the conclusion that our marriage was doomed because we weren't sexually compatible and I wondered how I, an intelligent and sexy modern woman, could have got myself into such a sad situation. I was afraid of losing this precious family unit we had built together and scared that if I was honest about our sexual differences that to stay in such a relationship would be to the detriment of my personal strength and modern womanhood. Didn't we deserve to have it all now and weren't we settling for less if we didn't demand the best? Well, isn't that a noose around the neck for marriage—especially when it seems that desire changes and negotiations are inevitable!

Writing the diaries helped Phoebe to focus more honestly on her own behaviour, and observe more carefully what was going on with her husband, Larry:

> I have taken deep breaths and held my tongue when L has driven me crazy. I have tried to be objective about my own games and habits—including saying no instead of maybe, putting distance between us as punishment (only hurts me more, duh!). I have watched and listened to L more accurately, looking to see who the real man is, noting his real feelings and looking at how he expresses himself and learning that often his anger or silence is his reaction to hurt or sadness. We've both

let our guards down more because I have stopped attacking him when I feel threatened (emotionally speaking) and I have calmly explained to him when I don't like his actions and have gained more respect from him and from my own self. Oh yes, it has been a journey.

She wrote the diaries on her own—she never even told Larry she was participating in the project. But it gave her the courage to talk more openly with him:

I have just kept on pushing the envelope, sitting down for yet another talk instead of being passive-aggressive. And it has started to pay off. At first it didn't feel natural, I felt I was trying hard to like and love someone whom perhaps I just didn't like—but then now and again, there was a glimmer of a new relationship—a friendship. Sexually, I stopped focusing on my wish list and what I thought I was missing out on and started looking at what I had that was good—someone warm to cuddle who smelt nice and who I was beginning to trust with my feelings again.

In her final letter to me, Phoebe shows what a difference this has made:

We had sex this morning—I was tired and I didn't have an orgasm, but I made myself ... look at the happiness on his face and see it not as sad because I wasn't passionate enough but see it as good that he can be happy and I am being close to him. And in turn, he cuddled me as we went back to sleep and told me that he loved me—that can't be so bad can it? So I say, all those bloody magazines and movies about hot sex and soul mates and happy-ever-after have got a lot to answer for. I have chosen a family, stability and kindness over passion, excitement and being 'hot'. I don't expect perfection any more but I don't feel hard done by. I did take some time to grieve the loss of my romantic dreams but it is better to live in the real world.

Of course, not everyone reached such peaceful compromise. Some of my diarists battled hard to open up communication with their partners, and ultimately got nowhere—some even dropped out of the research and a handful reported that their relationships had broken up. Here's Craig, reporting from Cairns:

> Nothing has changed with my situation though. My wife is still totally unresponsive, despite my best efforts to improve the conditions that might generate the symptoms. Any suggestion of ANY form of intimacy is shrugged off, or, more commonly, aggressively pushed away. In the end you realise that when you can't even get a passionate kiss (no tongues, just a nice peck or lasting embrace) then any other form of intimacy is definitely off the menu!! Even just trying to cuddle up beside her in bed on one cold night (with no sexual overtones—just an arm draped around her) was received with criticism that 'You were all over me last night'.

During the project, Craig tried hard to find a way to break through to his wife:

> Since our conversations began, I have tried being more genu-inely understanding and attentive but I suppose sometimes you just have to accept that the love/lust which was once there is no longer around and I no longer have the right fuel for the fire. I took a chance a few weeks back. I had really gone all out for my wife's birthday (as I always do) to make sure that she really had a good day (which I know she did) and for a change she was really relaxed and friendly and talkative, having been wined, dined and had a great family day out together. Everything was perfect and we were returning by train home with the kids, when she asked me what I wanted for my birthday (I usually get a T-shirt every year—sigh!!!). I replied that what I wanted more than anything was her (emotional) love, to which I got a cold reception and a response that it had to be earnt.

> After hearing my wife's comments on the train, I realised
> that this relationship is all about her needs and no consideration
> of mine. She has also done a lot that has also adversely affected
> the relationship but does not seem willing or able to accept that
> responsibility and puts all blame onto me. I have become more
> open and candid with my comments to her on the situation
> over the past twelve months and more honest about how I am
> feeling. Although this has not helped resolve the situation it
> has helped me gain back a bit of my self-esteem in that I feel
> I have finally grown some balls and can recognise that my own
> needs should be considered on a par with hers.

He's not feeling optimistic about their future together: 'I have
reached the stage that I will be putting the ultimatum that she
makes a decision about where she wants our relationship to go:
If she wants it to work, then let's make some changes in our
attitudes and circumstances and let's give it our best shot'.

It's unlikely their relationship will improve without that mutual
commitment to making it work. Fortunately, there's plenty of help
available for those who are keen to achieve change. There are
good self-help books, like Rosie King's *Good Loving, Great Sex*,
Michele Weiner Davis's *The Sex-starved Marriage* and Sandra
Pertot's *Perfectly Normal: Living and Loving with Low Libido*.[4]
Counselling may help too, although you do need to find someone
who is knowledgeable about both relationship and sexual counselling. (You can log on to my website—www.bettinaarndt.com.au—
to see my latest project.)

Then there's my sex diary approach.[5] Many of my sex-starved
diarists reported an improvement in sexual frequency—writing
sex diaries put sex on the agenda and that made a difference.
Many women were willing to explore the 'just do it' idea and found
that they enjoyed sex more when they took the initiative, making
their move when the moment was right for *them*. Of course, we

need to think about what exactly is the 'it' being talked about here. 'I'm not sure what "it" is that women should just do', writes David from Melbourne, making the point that 'it' needn't be intercourse. There's nothing wrong with 'outercourse', he suggests—using hands and lips to give pleasure, rather than assuming that coitus always has to be on the menu. It works a lot better for many of my female diarists to sometimes offer a hand job or oral sex when they are not in the mood for bonking.

It was striking that there were women who had never even considered having sex when they weren't in the mood—some reported it came as a relief to discover that they could respond provided they got their heads into the right place. But there were others who found that the 'just do it' idea still rankled. They couldn't shake off the lasting legacy of the message that in the absence of a burning desire for sex, they must say 'no'. When they felt let down or resentful about other aspects of the relationship, sexual generosity was rarely forthcoming.

'Desire might be a decision but is it a decision you really want to make?' asks Lucy. She says it all depends on what's happening in the relationship, grumbling that maybe this is just a new version of the 'think of England' model. Her response to the idea depends on how she is being treated: 'When I feel good about myself I feel strong and empowered—a more sexual being. If I'm constantly being corrected or put down, then there's not a lot of incentive for me to do anybody any "favours"'.

But Monica is the one who really reacted badly to the whole notion of 'just do it'. She's the woman I spoke about in Chapter 7 who has been living in a celibate marriage for the last three years, ever since she decided she could not face sex any more. 'I have been *just doing it* for many years—our marriage is now in a post "just do it" phase!' she says. Now, the very thought of the idea gets her knickers in a twist:

I hate this idea! Why the hell should women *just do it* when they have no desire? They are the ones who have to put up with the cold slime dripping between their legs, the urine infections, the fungal infections, the pain caused by dry mucosa, the tedium of the whole business. Just doing it is a great concept when you're young and can have a quickie while the kettle boils, but just doing it is a bit of an ordeal when you're forty plus and the juices have dried up.

Monica makes a passionate case, saying that the whole argument about accommodating men's desire is misguided:

I feel a tad let down that you're just urging women to do what they've been doing for years and, worse, applauding the possibility of medication to give women a chemical turn on which surely is essentially dishonest. The sexual mismatch is nothing new yet you're treating it as something urgent that must be addressed immediately. It seems simple really—our female bodies are there so that we can have children. When menopause comes along our function is complete and most of us are content to get on with it. Why oh why must we be TREATED with a pill for what is deemed to be physiologically normal? I feel strongly about this. There is nothing wrong with me so why must I be treated as if I am the abnormal one? If women must be treated for a low libido, why can't men be treated for their higher libido?

Yes, the sexual mismatch isn't new. But we live in an era of heightened expectations, where women are pushing an agenda of change, seeking what *they* want from their relationships. Women's list of demands is endless: more intimacy, more talk, closeness, shared household chores, greater sensitivity—even access to his innermost thoughts and feelings, for heaven's sake. It is not 'normal' or easy for men to suddenly start talking about feelings, regurgitating their emotions—yet this is what we are expecting them to do. In this context, it seems blatantly unfair to ignore the number one desire on many men's agendas—for more sex. How can we justify simply shutting up shop or forcing a man into a life spent grovelling for sex?

Yet it is easy to see the appeal of trying to get men to back off. There's an amusing chapter in Joan Sewell's book *I'd Rather Eat Chocolate* where she presents her ideal Oprah show, with the guests stars being men whose high sex drive is endangering their marriages. 'Men everywhere are now coming forward to reveal a very embarrassing secret: their obsessive need for sex. Afraid that their wives will leave them, men are now seeking help with ways to lower their libido', her fantasy Oprah proclaims, before trotting out the experts who offer hope for these men—in the form of an 'estrogen supplement' which only occasionally has the unfortunate side effect of giving men breasts. 'Why aren't men going out in droves to accommodate the lower sex drive of women rather than women always accommodating the higher sex drive of men', Sewell asks plaintively.[6]

Well, from what my sex diarists tell me, there are plenty of men doing the accommodating at the moment. Remember David Schnarch's pearl of wisdom about the lower drive partner being the one who sets the pace for sexual frequency?[7] It seems to me that the sexual tempo in most bedrooms is being slowed by women saying 'no', despite all the efforts of their partners to liven up the pace.

Yes, there are men, like Monica's husband, Greg, who decide that the rewards in their comfortable yet sexless marriage are sufficient, and that's fine. 'Greg adores me. I am sure he is saddened by the lack of love in our marriage but staying together is the least worst option for both of us', says Monica, stressing how well they get on and their mutual devotion to their three adult children. It helps that for many men, the sexual interest tends to diminish.

I remember talking to a friend in his fifties who had spent his life feeling driven by his strong sexual appetite. 'The monkey's got off my back', he told me, surprised to discover that sex was no longer such a big deal in his life.

But when a man—or indeed a woman—wants to be wanted, yearns to see lust in their partner's eyes, longs for the ultimate connection that lovemaking can provide, then this is a basic need that should not be ignored. Very few relationships can weather the devastating effects of constant rejection. Men spend their lives fearing rejection, says Sam, the Brisbane man from Chapter 1 who wrote so eloquently about sexual needs and mutual caring:

> Boys innately practice 'rejection training' and many men spend a lot of time managing their lives in such a way as to avoid being rebuffed. Eventually each man finds a woman with whom he can relax: one who obviously enjoys sex as much as he does; someone who accepts and loves him; someone who does not reject him. And so they are wed. Soon after, this woman decides to put her man on short rations: she rejects his advances. To a man it is devastating to be turned down by the very woman he chose because, at least in a large part, he thought he had no need to fear her rejection. Men are nowhere near as emotionally tough as we would like others to believe.

The sex diaries helped couples to understand that male vulnerability, and why sex is so important to men. But, equally so, the men came to realise that women's low drive does seem to be grounded in their biology, rather than being a rejection of their partners or a sign of declining love or interest. That made a real difference, explains Margaret from Melbourne: 'Our differences in desire have been a source of frustration, resentment and reduction of intimacy. And because of our belief that these differences were insurmountable and a serious sin of incompatibility, they have often resulted in a chasm between us that at times has felt unbreachable'.

That has now changed for Margaret and her husband, David:

> We now know that not only is such a difference common, it is normal. And we are learning to accommodate it. We are not failures. The most significant development that has come about since we made contact with you is my feeling that at last David has accepted that my sex drive and pleasure are much less than his and that's OK. My lack of interest doesn't mean I love him less than when I was hungry for sex before we married or that he needs to improve his techniques to get me excited. We are now satisfied to give each other the pleasure that we know the other enjoys without feeling put upon or resentful. Our sex life is now mutual rather than at odds with each other.

And the strangest thing of all, writes David, is, now that Margaret feels he is more accepting of who she is sexually, she is starting to change: 'It seems to have freed her to change to be more responsive sexually. This is the paradox—that acceptance can lead to change'.

Acceptance is the key to it all. Understanding why men's and women's sexual needs are different. And talking about it. Communicating about what you both want and why. Knowing that change is possible but that it comes from within—from moving on from blame and resentment to the acceptance of your partner as he or she is, and focusing on what *you* can do to make a difference. We all need to take responsibility for creating a joyful partnership where lovemaking is just one of the many ways of showing you care for each other. The desire to desire is where it all begins.

'Eroticism in the home requires active engagement and willful intent', writes Esther Perel, stressing the sense of playfulness that distinguishes couples who remain sensually alive to each other.[8] So many of my diarists are doing just that, seeing seduction as an end in itself, rejoicing in the erotic while delighting in its irreverence. It is that shared intention that allows them to bask in the comfort of love while still enjoying the heat of passion. They reap the rewards.

Notes

1 Fifty Thrusts and Don't Jiggle My Book

1 'Security Bad News for Sex Drive', BBC News, 14 August 2006, http://news.bbc.co.uk/2/hi/health/4790313.stm, viewed September 2008.
2 All names and some other personal details have been changed to protect the privacy of the diarists. These people were all volunteers, which introduces an obvious bias to the research. Only the brave are likely to put themselves forward for such a project. But luckily the group ended up including a remarkable range of people who represented many of the normal variations in desire patterns. The intention was never to obtain a representative survey but, rather, to focus on the rich personal stories that emerged through the diary process.
3 Shere Hite, *The Hite Report on Male Sexuality*, Alfred Knopf, New York, 1981.
4 Betty Friedan, *The Feminine Mystique*, WW Norton and Co., New York, 1963.
5 Fred Small, 'Pornography and Censorship', in Michael S Kimmel (ed.), *Men Confront Pornography*, Meridian, New York, 1990.
6 Nigel Marsh, *Fat, Forty and Fired*, Bantam, Sydney, 2005.
7 Nigel Marsh, *Observations of a Very Short Man*, Allen and Unwin, Sydney, 2007.
8 M Scott Peck, *The Road Less Travelled*, Touchstone, Clearwater, Florida, 2003.

2 Shifting the Sprinkler and Other Green Square Days

1 Esther Perel, *Mating in Captivity*, HarperCollins, New York, 2006.
2 Joan Sewell, *I'd Rather Eat Chocolate: Learning to Love My Low Libido*, Broadway Books, New York, 2007.
3 *The Sex Diaries* focuses only on heterosexual couples because it seemed impossible to include sufficient gay and lesbian couples in the research group to do justice to the complexities of homosexual relationships. There is already a considerable body of literature focusing on gay and lesbian sex lives—see the 'Lesbian Bed Death' box on page 21.
4 Janet Lever, 'The 1995 Advocate Survey of Sexuality and Relationships: The Women', *Advocate*, nos 687–8, 22 August 1995, pp. 22–30.
5 Philip Blumstein and Pepper Schwartz, *American Couples: Money, Work, Sex*, Morrow, New York, 1983.

6   Juliet Richters, 'Researching Sex between Women', paper given at 18th Congress of World Association for Sexual Health, 15–19 April 2007, www. worldsexology.org/doc/Abstract_Book_Sydney.pdf, viewed September 2008.
7   Suzanne Iasenza, 'The Big Lie: Lesbian Bed Death', *Family*, April 1999.
8   Richters.
9   Letitia Anne Peplau, Adam Fingerhut and Kristin P Beals, 'Sexuality in the Relationships of Lesbians and Gay Men', in John H Harvey, Amy Wenzel and Susan Sprecher (eds), *The Handbook of Sexuality in Close Relationships*, Lawrence Erlbaum Associates, Mahwah, NJ, 2004.
10 Blumstein and Schwartz.
11 Sandra Tsing Loh, 'She's Just Not That into You', *Atlantic Monthly*, March 2007, www.theatlantic.com/doc/200703/loh-libido, viewed September 2008.

3 Where Has She Gone, This Lover I Married?

1   Michael Gurian, *What Could He Be Thinking? A Guide to the Mysteries of a Man's Mind*, HarperCollins, London, 2003.
2   David Schnarch, *Passionate Marriage*, WW Norton and Co., New York, 1997.
3   Hugh Mackay, *Reinventing Australia*, HarperCollins, Sydney, 1993.
4   M Brinig and A Douglas, 'These Boots Are Made for Walking: Why Most Divorce Filers Are Women', *American Journal of Law and Economics*, vol. 2, 2000, pp. 126–69; Lixia Qu, Australian Institute of Family Studies (AIFS), pers. comm., September 2008, citing Ilene Wolcott and Jody Hughes, 'Towards Understanding the Reasons for Divorce', working paper no. 20, AIFS, Melbourne, June 1999, pp. 14–15.
5   Scott Haltzman, *The Secrets of Happily Married Men*, A Wiley, San Francisco, 2006.
6   Lillian Rubin, *Intimate Strangers: Men and Women Together*, Perennial Press, New York, 1984.
7   Ken Dempsey, *Inequalities in Marriage: Australia and Beyond*, Oxford University Press, Melbourne, 1997.
8   John M Gottman and Nan Silver, 'Principle 4: Let Your Partner Influence You', in *The Seven Principles for Making Marriages Work*, Three Rivers Press, New York, 1999.
9   Kate Grenville, *The Idea of Perfection*, Macmillan, Sydney, 1999.

4 The Search for the Elusive Pink Viagra

1   Juliet Richters and Chris Rissel, *Doing It Down Under: The Sexual Lives of Australians*, Allen and Unwin, Sydney, 2005.
2   Natalie Angier, *Woman: An Intimate Geography*, Houghton Mifflin Books, Boston, 1999.
3   Helen Fisher, *Why We Love: The Nature and Chemistry of Romantic Love*, Henry Holt and Co., New York, 2004.
4   Helen Fisher, *The Anatomy of Love: A Natural History of Adultery, Monogamy and Divorce*, Simon and Schuster, London, 1992.
5   Rosie King, *Good Loving, Great Sex*, Random House, Sydney, 1997.

6   Beatrice Faust, *Women, Sex and Pornography*, Penguin Books, Melbourne, 1980.
7   Alfred Charles Kinsey, Wardell B Pomeroy and Clyde E Martin, *Sexual Behavior in the Human Male*, WB Saunders Co., Philadelphia and London, 1948.
8   Michael Brezsnyak and Mark A Whisman, 'Sexual Desire and Relationship Functioning: The Effects of Marital Satisfaction and Power', *Journal of Sex and Marital Therapy*, vol. 30, no. 3, 2004, pp. 199–217.
9   Lillian Rubin, *Intimate Strangers: Men and Women Together*, Perennial Press, New York, 1984.
10 Michael Gurian, *What Could He Be Thinking? A Guide to the Mysteries of a Man's Mind*, HarperCollins, London, 2003.
11 Richters and Rissel.
12 Richard D Hayes, Catherine M Bennett, Christopher K Fairley and Lorraine Dennerstein, 'What Can Prevalence Studies Tell Us about Female Sexual Difficulty and Dysfunction?', *Journal of Sex and Marital Therapy*, vol. 3, no. 4, 2006, pp. 589–95.
13 Lorraine Dennerstein, Janet R Guthrie, Richard D Hayes, Leonard R DeRogatis and Philippe Lehert, 'Sexual Function, Dysfunction and Sexual Distress in a Prospective, Population-based Sample of Mid-aged, Australian-born Women', *Journal of Sex and Medicine*, forthcoming.
14 Ray Moynihan, 'The Marketing of a Disease: Female Sexual Dysfunction', *British Medical Journal*, no. 330, 22 January 2005, pp. 192–4.
15 Leonore Tiefer, *Sex Is Not a Natural Act and Other Essays*, Westview Press, Boulder, CO, 1995.
16 James Burleigh, 'Viagra Flops for Brainy Women', *Independent*, 1 March 2004.
17 Rebecca Urban, 'Rough Ride to Smooth Wrinkles', *Age*, 22 May 2004.
18 Michael Castleman, 'The ArginMax Effect', Salon.com, 28 November 2001, http://archive.salon.com/sex/feature/2001/12/05/arginmax/index.html, viewed September 2008.
19 Monash University, 'Testosterone and Androgens in Women', Women's Health Program, 15 March 2005, http://womenshealth.med.monash.edu.au/documents/testosterone-in-women.pdf, viewed September 2008.
20 Susan Davis et al., 'Safety and Efficacy of a Testosterone Metered-dose Transdermal Spray for Treating Decreased Sexual Satisfaction in Premenopausal Women', *Annals of Internal Medicine*, vol. 148, no. 8, 15 April 2008, pp. 569–77.
21 ibid.
22 Margaret Redelman, pers. comm., April 2004.
23 ibid.
24 In her book *Bonk*, Mary Roach describes two likely prospects. One is bremelanotide, nicknamed 'the Barbie drug' because it stimulates the cells that cause skin to tan, suppresses appetite and ups libido. Then there's a central nervous system drug called flibanserin, which was originally tested as an antidepressant. See Mary Roach, *Bonk: The Curious Coupling of Sex and Science*, Text Publishing, Melbourne, 2008.

25   Gemma O'Brien, School of Biological, Biomedical and Molecular Sciences, University of New England, pers. comm., March 2008.

26   Kate M Dunn, Lynn F Cherkas and Tim D Spector, 'Genetic Influences on Variation in Female Orgasmic Function', *Biological Letters*, vol. 1, 2005, pp. 260–5; SV Glinianaia, J Rankin and C Wright, 'Congenital Anomalies in Twins: A Register-based Study', *Human Reproduction*, vol. 23, 2008, pp. 1306–11.

27   Gemma O'Brien.

28   Dennerstein et al.

29   Susan Davis, 'The Effects of Tibolone on Mood and Libido', *Menopause*, vol. 9, no. 3, May 2002, pp. 162–70.

30   Dennerstein et al.

5   Just Do It!

1   Helen S Kaplan, 'Hypoactive Sexual Desire', *Journal of Sex and Marital Therapy*, vol. 3, no. 1, spring 1977, pp. 3–9.

2   *R v. Johns*, Supreme Court, SA No. SCCRM/91/452, 26 August 1992.

3   Rosemary Basson, 'Sexual Desire and Arousal Disorders in Women', *New England Journal of Medicine*, vol. 354, no. 14, April 2006, pp. 1497–506.

4   Much has been made of a study of nurses by Michael Sands from the University of Western Ontario in Canada; see Michael Sands and William Fisher, 'Women's Endorsement of Models of Female Sexual Response', *Journal of Sexual Medicine*, vol. 4, 2007, pp. 708–19. With his German colleague William Fisher, Sands asked nurses which model of sexual functioning most reflected their own experience. The researchers found about one third of women said their response fitted the Basson model, where they often engaged in sex for reasons other than their own desire. But Sands also found that these women were among those most likely to have sexual concerns—'reflective of women who experience more problematic, unsatisfying sexual response'. That makes sense—women who don't experience much sexual desire are often unhappy about their low libido. But this doesn't mean that Basson's model can be dismissed as applying only to sexual misfits. While Basson found that only one third reported this pattern, some much larger studies found that a majority of women report a low sex drive. So while there are plenty of women whose sexual response is driven by their own desire, for just as many women, if not more, the Basson model is a better fit.

5   Michele Weiner Davis, *The Sex-starved Marriage*, Simon and Schuster, London, 2003.

6   Bettina Arndt, 'Where's Our Pink Viagra?', *Australian Women's Weekly*, June 2004.

7   Caitlin Flanagan, 'The Wifely Duty', *Atlantic Monthly*, vol. 291, no. 1, January– February 2003, pp. 171–81.

8   ibid.

9   blue milk, 'Sex to Save the Family', 28 July 2007, http://bluemilk.wordpress. com/2007/07/28/sex-to-save-the-family, viewed September 2008.

10 Basson.
11 Charla Muller and Betsy Thorpe, 365 *Nights: A Memoir of Intimacy*, Berkley Books, New York, 2008.
12 The Mullers aren't the only couple who have recently written about their private sex marathon. Douglas Brown, a 42-year-old reporter at *The Denver Post*, gives an entertaining account of 101 consecutive days of sex with his wife, Annie, in his book *Just Do It*. Here, too, the couple's goal was to spice up their sex lives, a task which they pursued with a vengeance. A far more adventurous and more sexually compatible couple than the Mullers, the Browns happily bonk their way through a cold Colorado winter, spicing things up by visiting a sex expo, learning 'hot' yoga to get limber and experimenting with all manner of sex toys. Like the Mullers, the surprise was in how much closer it brought them, as they found themselves relishing deeper conversations, holding hands and becoming more aware of each other, emotionally and physically. See Douglas Brown, *Just Do It*, Crown, New York, 2008.

6 Juicy Tomatoes and the Celery Stick Men

1 Joan Sewell, *I'd Rather Eat Chocolate: Learning to Love My Low Libido*, Broadway Books, New York, 2007. For the interview, see Sara Lipka, 'Not Tonight Dear', The Atlantic.com, 6 February 2007, www.theatlantic.com/doc/200702u/no-sex, viewed September 2008.
2 Juliet Richters and Chris Rissel, *Doing It Down Under: The Sexual Lives of Australians*, Allen and Unwin, Sydney, 2005.
3 Michele Weiner Davis, *The Sex-starved Wife: What to Do When He's Lost Desire*, Simon and Schuster, New York, 2008.
4 Michele Weiner Davis, *The Sex-starved Marriage*, Simon and Schuster, London, 2003.
5 EJH Meuleman and JJDM van Lankveld, 'Hypoactive Sexual Desire Disorder: An Underestimated Condition in Men', *BJU International*, vol. 95, no. 3, February 2005, pp. 291–6.
6 Richters and Rissel.
7 Bob Berkowitz and Susan Yager-Berkowitz, *He's Just Not Up for It Anymore: Why Men Stop Having Sex, and What You Can Do about It*, William Morrow, New York, 2008.
8 ibid.
9 Weiner Davis, *The Sex-starved Wife*.
10 Berkowitz and Yager-Berkowitz.
11 'Tom', 'Getting Back in the Game: Impotency, PCa and the Single Man', Phoenix 5, March 2000, www.phoenix5.org/stories/firstpers/perstomimpot.html.
12 Weiner Davis, *The Sex-starved Wife*.
13 ibid.
14 ibid.
15 ibid.
16 ibid.

17 Weiner Davis, *The Sex-starved Marriage*.
18 Esther Perel, *Mating in Captivity*, HarperCollins, New York, 2006.

7 The World's Most Boring Affair

1   Eric R Widmer, Judith Treas and Robert Newcomb, 'Attitudes Towards Non-marital Sex in 24 Countries', *Journal of Sex Research*, November 1998, pp. 349–58.
2   Juliet Richters and Chris Rissel, *Doing It Down Under: The Sexual Lives of Australians*, Allen and Unwin, Sydney, 2005.
3   Elizabeth Bowen, *The House in Paris*, Alfred A Knopf, New York, 1935.
4   Annette Lawson, *Adultery: An Analysis of Love and Betrayal*, Basic Books, New York, 1998.
5   Richters and Rissel.
6   'Voice of Australian Women', *Australian Women's Weekly*, April 2008.
7   Juliet Richters, pers. comm., September 2008.
8   Richters and Rissel.
9   Shirley Glass, 'Shattered Vows: Getting beyond Betrayal', *Psychology Today*, July–August 1998.
10 Pamela Druckerman, *Lust in Translation: Infidelity from Tokyo to Tennessee*, Penguin, London, 2007.
11 Esther Perel, *Mating in Captivity*, HarperCollins, New York, 2006.
12 ibid.
13 Heidi Greiling and David M Buss, 'Women's Sexual Strategies: The Hidden Dimension of Extrapair Mating', *Personality and Individual Differences*, vol. 28, 2000, pp. 929–63.

8 Two Pounds of Liver and a Cabbage

1   David Schnarch, *Passionate Marriage*, WW Norton and Co., New York, 1997.

9 Laundry Gets You Laid?

1   John Gottman, *Why Marriages Succeed or Fail and How You Can Make Yours Last*, Simon and Schuster, New York, 1994.
2   Neil Chethik, *VoiceMale: What Husbands Really Think about Their Marriages, Their Wives, Sex, Housework, and Commitment*, Simon and Schuster, New York, 2006.
3   Dan Savage, 'Savage Love', The AV Club, 14 March 2007, www.avclub.com/content/savage/mar-14-2007_0, viewed September 2008.
4   Joan Sewell, *I'd Rather Eat Chocolate: Learning to Love My Low Libido*, Broadway Books, New York, 2007.
5   Savage.
6   Michele Weiner Davis, *The Sex-starved Marriage*, Simon and Schuster, London, 2003.
7   Ken Dempsey, *Inequalities in Marriage: Australia and Beyond*, Oxford University Press, Melbourne, 1997.

10   Get That Thing Away from Me!

1   Harriet Lerner, *The Mother Dance*, HarperCollins, New York, 1999.
2   Kaalii Cargill, pers. comm., March 2008.
3   Anthony Pietropinto and Jacqueline Simenauer, *Not Tonight Dear: How to Reawaken Your Sexual Desire*, Doubleday, New York, 1990.
4   Sandra Pertot, *Perfectly Normal: Living and Loving with Low Libido*, Rodale, Emmaus, PA, 2005.
5   Esther Perel, *Mating in Captivity*, HarperCollins, New York, 2006.
6   ibid.
7   Sheila Kitzinger, *Ourselves as Mothers: The Universal Experience of Motherhood*, Addison-Wesley, Reading, PA, 1994.
8   Perel.
9   ibid.
10 Jenny Hislop and Sara Arber, 'Sleepers Wake! The Gendered Nature of Sleep Disruption among Mid-life Women', *Sociology*, vol. 37, no. 4, 2003, pp. 695–711.
11 ibid.
12 Daniel G Amen, *Sex on the Brain*, Three Rivers Press, New York, 2007.

11   Blind Man in the Dark Trying to Find a Black Cat

1   Irma Kurtz, *Beds of Nails and Roses: Witty Observations on Enjoying Life as a Modern Woman*, Dodd, Mead, New York, 1983.
2   Lionel Shriver, *The Post-birthday World*, HarperCollins, New York, 2007.
3   ibid.
4   Leonore Tiefer, *Sex Is Not a Natural Act and Other Essays*, Westview Press, Boulder, CO, 1995, p. 178.
5   Joan Sewell, *I'd Rather Eat Chocolate: Learning to Love My Low Libido*, Broadway Books, New York, 2007.
6   ibid. Even women with very low sex drives report that they sometimes masturbate. They masturbate when *they* have the urge—particularly when using a vibrator, they know it is quick, easy and guarantees results. That's a very different experience from putting out for a partner. But there are also women who simply aren't interested. 'I am forty-four years old and have masturbated twice in my life. It's not that I think it's wrong or dirty, I just never have had the desire', reports another diarist. The *Sex in Australia* Survey found that 65 per cent of men and 35 per cent of women reported masturbating in the past year; see Juliet Richters and Chris Rissel, *Doing It Down Under: The Sexual Lives of Australians*, Allen and Unwin, Sydney, 2005.
7   Sewell.
8   ibid.
9   Marcia Douglass and Lisa Douglass, *Are We Having Fun Yet? The Intelligent Woman's Guide to Sex*, Hyperion, New York, 1997.
10 Richters and Rissel.
11 Alex Comfort, *The Joy of Sex: A Gourmet Guide to Lovemaking*, Simon and Schuster, New York, 1972.

12 Ian Kerner, *She Comes First: The Thinking Man's Guide to Pleasuring a Woman*, HarperCollins, New York, 2004.

13 John Perry, 'The Primitive Psychology of Alfred Kinsey', paper presented at Spring Scientific Meeting of the Maine Psychological Association, Bates College, Lewiston, ME, 1984, www.incontinet.com/kinsey.htm, viewed September 2008.

14 Catherine Blackledge, *The Story of V: Opening Pandora's Box*, Weidenfeld and Nicolson, London, 2003.

15 Germaine Greer, *The Female Eunuch*, Macgibbon and Kee Limited, London, 1970.

16 Shere Hite, *The Hite Report: A Nationwide Study of Female Sexuality*, Macmillan, New York, 1976.

17 Andrea Dworkin, *Intercourse*, Free Press, New York, 1988.

18 Mary Roach, in her book *Bonk*, gives a hilarious description not only of the work of these Dutch scientists, but also of her own first-hand experience, of bonking gently with her husband within the confines of an MRI; see Mary Roach, *Bonk: The Curious Coupling of Sex and Science*, Text Publishing, Melbourne, 2008.

19 Helen E O'Connell, John M Hutson, Colin R Anderson and Robert J Plenter, 'Anatomical Relationship between Urethra and Clitoris', *Journal of Urology*, vol. 159, no. 6, 1998, pp. 1892–7.

20 Barry Komisaruk, Carlos Beyer-Flores and Beverly Whipple, *The Science of Orgasm*, Johns Hopkins University Press, Baltimore, 2006.

21 Blackledge.

22 Sigmund Freud, *Three Essays on the Theory of Sexuality*, trans. James Strachey, Basic Books, New York, 1962 [1905].

23 Roach.

24 Stuart Brody, Ellen Laan and Rik Van Lunsen, 'Concordance between Women's Physiological and Subjective Sexual Arousal Is Associated with Consistency of Orgasm during Intercourse but Not Other Sexual Behavior', *Journal of Sex and Marital Therapy*, vol. 29, 2003, pp. 15–23.

25 Brody's most recent work has found that women who don't climax vaginally are more prone to a range of psychological problems—social anxiety, depression and so on. Stuart Brody and Rui M Costa, 'Vaginal Orgasm Is Associated with Less Use of Immature Psychological Defense Mechanisms', *Journal of Sexual Medicine*, vol. 5, no. 5, May 2008, pp. 1167–76.

26 As Mary Roach explains in her book *Bonk*, Kinsey concluded that the most important factor determining whether a woman climaxes during intercourse is 'one's level of engagement in the proceedings'. Women often are more likely to climax when they are 'on top', Kinsey explained, because less inhibited women are more likely to use such a position and, in doing so, they have more control over speed, depth and direction.

27 Kate M Dunn, Lynn F Cherkas and Tim D Spector, 'Genetic Influences on Variation in Female Orgasmic Function', *Biological Letters*, vol. 1, 2005, pp. 260–5; SV Glinianaia, J Rankin and C Wright, 'Congenital Anomalies in Twins: A Register-based Study', *Human Reproduction*, vol. 23, 2008, pp. 1306–11; Juliette M Harris, Lynn F Cherkas, Bernet S Kato, Julia R Heiman and

Tim D Spector, 'Normal Variations in Personality Are Associated with Coital Orgasmic Frequency in Heterosexual Women: A Population-based Study', *Journal of Sexual Medicine*, vol. 5, 2008, pp. 1177–83.

28   Khytam Dawood, Katherine M Kirk, J Michael Bailey, Paul W Andrews and Nicholas G Martin, 'Genetic and Environmental Influences on the Frequency of Orgasm in Women', *Twin Research and Human Genetics*, vol. 8, no. 1, January 2005, pp. 27–33.

29   Eric W Corty and Jenay M Guardiani, 'Canadian and American Sex Therapists' Perceptions of Normal and Abnormal Ejaculatory Latencies: How Long Should Intercourse Last?', *Journal of Sexual Medicine*, vol. 5, no. 5, May 2008, pp. 1251–6.

30   ibid.

31   Richters and Rissel.

32   David Schnarch, *Passionate Marriage*, WW Norton and Co., New York, 1997.

12   It's in His Kiss! That's Where It Is

1   Susan M Hughes, Marissa A Harrison and Gordon G Gallup, 'Sex Differences in Romantic Kissing among College Students: An Evolutionary Perspective', *Evolutionary Psychology*, vol. 5, no. 3, 2007, pp. 612–31.

13   Three Cheers for Mr Pinocchio

1   Alastair H MacLennan, Stephen P Myers and Anne W Taylor, 'The Continuing Use of Complementary and Alternative Medicine in South Australia: Costs and Beliefs in 2004', *Medical Journal of Australia*, vol. 184, no. 1, 2006, pp. 27–31.

2   Committee of Inquiry into Impotency Treatment Services, *The 1998 Report of the Ministerial Committee of Inquiry into Impotency Treatment Services in NSW*, Health Care Complaints Commission, Sydney, 1998.

3   Cully Carson and Chris G McMahon, *Fast Facts: Erectile Dysfunction*, Health Press, Oxford, 2008.

4   Agency for Health Care Research and Quality, 'Comparative Effectiveness of Therapies for Clinically Localized Prostate Cancer', Executive Summary, US Department of Health and Human Services, 5 February 2008, http://effectivehealthcare.ahrq.gov/healthInfo.cfm?infotype=rr&ProcessID=9&DocID=79, viewed September 2008.

5   'Sharon', 'Moving between the Phases', Phoenix 5, April 2000, www.phoenix5.org/stories/firstpers/perssharonemot.html.

6   Irma Kurtz, *Beds of Nails and Roses: Witty Observations on Enjoying Life as a Modern Woman*, Dodd, Mead, New York, 1983.

7   Rosie King, pers. comm., March 2008.

8   ibid.

9   ibid.

10 Bernie Zilbergeld, *The New Male Sexuality: The Truth about Men, Sex and Pleasure*, Bantam, New York, 1992.

11 ibid.

12   Julius Lester, 'Being a Boy', *Ms. Magazine*, June 1973, pp. 112–13.
13   David M Friedman, *A Mind of Its Own: A Cultural History of the Penis*, Robert Hale, London, 2003.

14 Bad Health, Thinking It Is Silly and No Bicycle

1   Alex Comfort, *The Joy of Sex: A Gourmet Guide to Lovemaking*, Simon and Schuster, New York, 1972.
2   beyondblue, www.beyondblue.org.au, viewed September 2008.
3   Helen Fisher, *The Anatomy of Love: A Natural History of Adultery, Monogamy and Divorce*, Simon and Schuster, London, 1992.
4   Michele Weiner Davis, *The Sex-starved Marriage*, Simon and Schuster, London, 2003.

15 The Desire to Desire

1   Helen Fisher, 'Helen Fisher on TEDTalks', TEDBlog, 6 September 2006, http://tedblog.typepad.com/tedblog/2006/09/helen_fisher_on.html, viewed September 2008.
2   Dietrich Klusman, 'Sexual Motivation and the Duration of Partnership', *Archives of Sexual Behaviour*, vol. 31, no. 3, pp. 275–87.
3   Lorraine Dennerstein, Janet R Guthrie, Richard D Hayes, Leonard R DeRogatis and Philippe Lehert, 'Sexual Function, Dysfunction and Sexual Distress in a Prospective, Population-based Sample of Mid-aged, Australian-born Women', *Journal of Sex and Medicine*, forthcoming.
4   Rosie King, *Good Loving, Great Sex*, Random House, Sydney, 1997; Michele Weiner Davis, *The Sex-starved Marriage*, Simon and Schuster, London, 2003; Sandra Pertot, *Perfectly Normal: Living and Loving with Low Libido*, Rodale, Emmaus, PA, 2005.
5   For details, see my website: www.bettinaarndt.com.au
6   Joan Sewell, *I'd Rather Eat Chocolate: Learning to Love My Low Libido*, Broadway Books, New York, 2007.
7   David Schnarch, *Passionate Marriage*, WW Norton and Co., New York, 1997.
8   Esther Perel, *Mating in Captivity*, HarperCollins, New York, 2006.

Bibliography

Agency for Health Care Research and Quality, 'Comparative Effectiveness of Therapies for Clinically Localized Prostate Cancer', Executive Summary, US Department of Health and Human Services, 5 February 2008, http://effectivehealthcare.ahrq.gov/healthInfo.cfm?infotype=rr&ProcessID=9&DocID=79, viewed September 2008.

Amen, Daniel G, *Sex on the Brain*, Three Rivers Press, New York, 2007.

Angier, Natalie, *Woman: An Intimate Geography*, Houghton Mifflin Books, Boston, 1999.

Arndt, Bettina, 'Where's Our Pink Viagra?', *Australian Women's Weekly*, June 2004.

Basson, Rosemary, 'Sexual Desire and Arousal Disorders in Women', *New England Journal of Medicine*, vol. 354, no. 14, April 2006, pp. 1497–506.

Berkowitz, Bob and Susan Yager-Berkowitz, *He's Just Not Up for It Anymore: Why Men Stop Having Sex, and What You Can Do about It*, William Morrow, New York, 2008.

beyondblue, www.beyondblue.org.au, viewed September 2008.

Blackledge, Catherine, *The Story of V: Opening Pandora's Box*, Weidenfeld and Nicolson, London, 2003.

blue milk, 'Sex to Save the Family', 28 July 2007, http://bluemilk.wordpress.com/2007/07/28/sex-to-save-the-family, viewed September 2008.

Blumstein, Philip and Pepper Schwartz, *American Couples: Money, Work, Sex*, Morrow, New York, 1983.

Bowen, Elizabeth, *The House in Paris*, Alfred A Knopf, New York, 1935.

Brezsnyak, Michael and Mark A Whisman, 'Sexual Desire and Relationship Functioning: The Effects of Marital Satisfaction and Power', *Journal of Sex and Marital Therapy*, vol. 30, no. 3, 2004, pp. 199–217.

Brinig, M and A Douglas, 'These Boots Are Made for Walking: Why Most Divorce Filers Are Women', *American Journal of Law and Economics*, vol. 2, 2000, pp. 126–69.

Brody, Stuart and Rui M Costa, 'Vaginal Orgasm Is Associated with Less Use of Immature Psychological Defense Mechanisms', *Journal of Sexual Medicine*, vol. 5, no. 5, May 2008, pp. 1167–76.

Brody, Stuart, Ellen Laan and Rik Van Lunsen, 'Concordance between Women's Physiological and Subjective Sexual Arousal Is Associated with Consistency of Orgasm during Intercourse but Not Other Sexual Behavior', *Journal of Sex and Marital Therapy*, vol. 29, 2003, pp. 15–23.

Brown, Douglas, *Just Do It*, Crown, New York, 2008.

Burleigh, James, 'Viagra Flops for Brainy Women', *Independent*, 1 March 2004.

Carson, Cully and Chris G McMahon, *Fast Facts: Erectile Dysfunction*, Health Press, Oxford, 2008.

Castleman, Michael, 'The ArginMax Effect', Salon.com, 28 November 2001, http://archive.salon.com/sex/feature/2001/12/05/arginmax/index.html, viewed September 2008.

Chethik, Neil, *VoiceMale: What Husbands Really Think about Their Marriages, Their Wives, Sex, Housework, and Commitment*, Simon and Schuster, New York, 2006.

Comfort, Alex, *The Joy of Sex: A Gourmet Guide to Lovemaking*, Simon and Schuster, New York, 1972.

Committee of Inquiry into Impotency Treatment Services, *The 1998 Report of the Ministerial Committee of Inquiry into Impotency Treatment Services in NSW*, Health Care Complaints Commission, Sydney, 1998.

Corty, Eric W and Jenay M Guardiani, 'Canadian and American Sex Therapists' Perceptions of Normal and Abnormal Ejaculatory Latencies: How Long Should Intercourse Last?', *Journal of Sexual Medicine*, vol. 5, no. 5, May 2008, pp. 1251–6.

Davis, Susan, 'The Effects of Tibolone on Mood and Libido, *Menopause*, vol. 9, no. 3, May 2002, pp. 162–70.

Davis, Susan, Mary-Anne Papalia, Robert Norman, Sheila O'Neill, Margaret Redelman, Margaret Williamson, Bronwyn GA Stuckey, John Wlodarczyk, Karen Gardner and Andrew Humberstone, 'Safety and Efficacy of a Testosterone Metered-dose Transdermal Spray for Treating Decreased Sexual Satisfaction in Premenopausal Women', *Annals of Internal Medicine*, vol. 148, no. 8, 15 April 2008, pp. 569–77.

Dawood, Khytam, Katherine M Kirk, J Michael Bailey, Paul W Andrews and Nicholas G Martin, 'Genetic and Environmental Influences on the Frequency of Orgasm in Women', *Twin Research and Human Genetics*, vol. 8, no. 1, January 2006, pp. 27–33.

Dempsey, Ken, *Inequalities in Marriage: Australia and Beyond*, Oxford University Press, Melbourne, 1997.

Dennerstein, Lorraine, Janet R Guthrie, Richard D Hayes, Leonard R DeRogatis and Philippe Lehert, 'Sexual Function, Dysfunction and Sexual Distress in a Prospective, Population-based Sample of Mid-aged, Australian-born Women', *Journal of Sex and Medicine*, forthcoming.

Douglass, Marcia and Lisa Douglass, *Are We Having Fun Yet? The Intelligent Woman's Guide to Sex*, Hyperion, New York, 1997.

Druckerman, Pamela, *Lust in Translation: Infidelity from Tokyo to Tennessee*, Penguin, London, 2007.

Dunn, Kate M, Lynn F Cherkas and Tim D Spector, 'Genetic Influences on Variation in Female Orgasmic Function', *Biological Letters*, vol. 1, 2005, pp. 260–5.

Dworkin, Andrea, *Intercourse*, Free Press, New York, 1988.

Faust, Beatrice, *Women, Sex and Pornography*, Penguin Books, Melbourne, 1980.

Fisher, Helen, *The Anatomy of Love: A Natural History of Adultery, Monogamy and Divorce*, Simon and Schuster, London, 1992.

——*Why We Love: The Nature and Chemistry of Romantic Love*, Henry Holt and Co., New York, 2004.

——'Helen Fisher on TEDTalks', TEDBlog, 6 September 2006, http://tedblog. type pad.com/tedblog/2006/09/helen_fisher_on.html, viewed September 2008.

Flanagan, Caitlin, 'The Wifely Duty', *Atlantic Monthly*, vol. 291, no. 1, January–February 2003, pp. 171–81.

Freud, Sigmund, *Three Essays on the Theory of Sexuality*, trans. James Strachey, Basic Books, New York, 1962 [1905].

Friedan, Betty, *The Feminine Mystique*, WW Norton and Co., New York, 1963.

Friedman, David M, *A Mind of Its Own: A Cultural History of the Penis*, Robert Hale, London, 2003.

Glass, Shirley, 'Shattered Vows: Getting beyond Betrayal', *Psychology Today*, July–August 1998.

Glinianaia, SV, J Rankin and C Wright, 'Congenital Anomalies in Twins: A Register-based Study', *Human Reproduction*, vol. 23, 2008, pp. 1306–11.

Gottman, John, *Why Marriages Succeed or Fail and How You Can Make Yours Last*, Simon and Schuster, New York, 1994.

Gottman, John M and Nan Silver, 'Principle 4: Let Your Partner Influence You', in *The Seven Principles for Making Marriages Work*, Three Rivers Press, New York, 1999.

Greer, Germaine, *The Female Eunuch*, Macgibbon and Kee Limited, London, 1970.

Greiling, Heidi and David M Buss, 'Women's Sexual Strategies: The Hidden Dimension of Extrapair Mating', *Personality and Individual Differences*, vol. 28, 2000, pp. 929–63.

Grenville, Kate, *The Idea of Perfection*, Macmillan, Sydney, 1999.

Gurian, Michael, *What Could He Be Thinking? A Guide to the Mysteries of a Man's Mind*, HarperCollins, London, 2003.

Haltzman, Scott, *The Secrets of Happily Married Men*, A Wiley, San Francisco, 2006.

Harris, Juliette M, Lynn F Cherkas, Bernet S Kato, Julia R Heiman and Tim D Spector, 'Normal Variations in Personality Are Associated with Coital Orgasmic Frequency in Heterosexual Women: A Population-based Study', *Journal of Sexual Medicine*, vol. 5, 2008, pp. 1177–83.

Hayes, Richard D, Catherine M Bennett, Christopher K Fairley and Lorraine Dennerstein, 'What Can Prevalence Studies Tell Us about Female Sexual Difficulty and Dysfunction?', *Journal of Sex and Marital Therapy*, vol. 3, no. 4, 2006, pp. 589–95.

Hislop, Jenny and Sara Arber, 'Sleepers Wake! The Gendered Nature of Sleep Disruption among Mid-life Women', *Sociology*, vol. 37, no. 4, 2003, pp. 695–711.

Hite, Shere, *The Hite Report: A Nationwide Study of Female Sexuality*, Macmillan, New York, 1976.

——*The Hite Report on Male Sexuality*, Alfred Knopf, New York, 1981.

Hughes Susan M, Marissa A Harrison and Gordon G Gallup, 'Sex Differences in Romantic Kissing among College Students: An Evolutionary Perspective', *Evolutionary Psychology*, vol. 5, no. 3, 2007, pp. 612–31.

Iasenza, Suzanne, 'The Big Lie: Lesbian Bed Death', *Family*, April 1999.

Kaplan, Helen S, 'Hypoactive Sexual Desire', *Journal of Sex and Marital Therapy*, vol. 3, no. 1, spring 1977, pp. 3–9.

Kerner, Ian, *She Comes First: The Thinking Man's Guide to Pleasuring a Woman*, HarperCollins, New York, 2004.

King, Rosie, *Good Loving, Great Sex*, Random House, Sydney, 1997.

Kinsey, Alfred Charles, Wardell B Pomeroy and Clyde E Martin, *Sexual Behavior in the Human Male*, WB Saunders Co., Philadelphia and London, 1948.

Kitzinger, Sheila, *Ourselves as Mothers: The Universal Experience of Motherhood*, Addison-Wesley, Reading, PA, 1994.

Klusman, Dietrich, 'Sexual Motivation and the Duration of Partnership', *Archives of Sexual Behaviour*, vol. 31, no. 3, pp. 275–87.

Komisaruk, Barry, Carlos Beyer-Flores and Beverly Whipple, *The Science of Orgasm*, Johns Hopkins University Press, Baltimore, 2006.

Kurtz, Irma, *Beds of Nails and Roses: Witty Observations on Enjoying Life as a Modern Woman*, Dodd, Mead, New York, 1983.

Lawson, Annette, *Adultery: An Analysis of Love and Betrayal*, Basic Books, New York, 1998.

Lerner, Harriet, *The Mother Dance*, HarperCollins, New York, 1999.

Lester, Julius, 'Being a Boy', *Ms. Magazine*, June 1973, pp. 112–13.

Lever, Janet, 'The 1995 Advocate Survey of Sexuality and Relationships: The Women', *Advocate*, nos 687–8, 22 August 1995, pp. 22–30.

Lipka, Sara, 'Not Tonight Dear', The Atlantic.com, 6 February 2007, www. theatlantic.com/doc/200702u/no-sex, viewed September 2008.

Mackay, Hugh, *Reinventing Australia*, HarperCollins, Sydney, 1993.

MacLennan, Alastair H, Stephen P Myers and Anne W Taylor, 'The Continuing Use of Complementary and Alternative Medicine in South Australia: Costs and Beliefs in 2004', *Medical Journal of Australia*, vol. 184, no. 1, 2006, pp. 27–31.

Marsh, Nigel, *Fat, Forty and Fired*, Bantam, Sydney, 2005.

——*Observations of a Very Short Man*, Allen and Unwin, Sydney, 2007.

Meuleman, EJH and JJDM van Lankveld, 'Hypoactive Sexual Desire Disorder: An Underestimated Condition in Men', *BJU International*, vol. 95, no. 3, February 2005, pp. 291–6.

Moynihan, Ray, 'The Marketing of a Disease: Female Sexual Dysfunction', *British Medical Journal*, no. 330, 22 January 2005, pp. 192–4.

Muller, Charla and Betsy Thorpe, 365 *Nights: A Memoir of Intimacy*, Berkley Books, New York, 2008.

O'Brien, Gemma, School of Biological, Biomedical and Molecular Sciences, University of New England, pers. comm., March 2008.

O'Connell, Helen E, John M Hutson, Colin R Anderson and Robert J Plenter, 'Anatomical Relationship between Urethra and Clitoris', *Journal of Urology*, vol. 159, no. 6, 1998, pp. 1892–7.

Peck, M Scott, *The Road Less Travelled*, Touchstone, Clearwater, Florida, 2003.

Peplau, Letitia Anne, Adam Fingerhut and Kristin P Beals, 'Sexuality in the Relationships of Lesbians and Gay Men', in John H Harvey, Amy Wenzel and Susan Sprecher (eds), *The Handbook of Sexuality in Close Relationships*, Lawrence Erlbaum Associates, Mahwah, NJ, 2004.

Perel, Esther, *Mating in Captivity*, HarperCollins, New York, 2006.

Perry, John, 'The Primitive Psychology of Alfred Kinsey', paper presented at Spring Scientific Meeting of the Maine Psychological Association, Bates College, Lewiston, ME, 1984, www.incontinet.com/kinsey.htm, viewed September 2008.

Pertot, Sandra, *Perfectly Normal: Living and Loving with Low Libido*, Rodale, Emmaus, PA, 2005.

Pietropinto, Anthony and Jacqueline Simenauer, *Not Tonight Dear: How to Reawaken Your Sexual Desire*, Doubleday, New York, 1990.

Qu, Lixia, Australian Institute of Family Studies (AIFS), pers. comm., September 2008.

R v. Johns, Supreme Court, SA No. SCCRM/91/452, 26 August 1992.

Richters, Juliet, 'Researching Sex between Women', paper given at 18th Congress of World Association for Sexual Health, 15–19 April 2007, www.worldsexology.org/doc/Abstract_Book_Sydney.pdf, viewed September 2008.

Richters, Juliet and Chris Rissel, *Doing It Down Under: The Sexual Lives of Australians*, Allen and Unwin, Sydney. 2005.

Roach, Mary, *Bonk: The Curious Coupling of Sex and Science*, Text Publishing, Melbourne, 2008.

Rubin, Lillian, *Intimate Strangers: Men and Women Together*, Perennial Press, New York, 1984.

Sands, Michael and William Fisher, 'Women's Endorsement of Models of Female Sexual Response', *Journal of Sexual Medicine*, vol. 4, 2007, pp. 708–9.

Savage, Dan, 'Savage Love', The AV Club, 14 March 2007, www.avclub.com/content/savage/mar-14-2007_0, viewed September 2008.

Schnarch, David, *Passionate Marriage*, WW Norton and Co., New York, 1997.

'Security Bad News for Sex Drive', BBC News, 14 August 2006, http://news.bbc.co.uk/2/hi/health/4790313.stm, viewed September 2008.

Sewell, Joan, *I'd Rather Eat Chocolate: Learning to Love My Low Libido*, Broadway Books, New York, 2007.

'Sharon', 'Moving between the Phases', Phoenix 5, April 2000, www.phoenix5.org/stories/firstpers/perssharonemot.html, viewed November 2008.

Shriver, Lionel, *The Post-birthday World*, HarperCollins, New York, 2007.

Small, Fred, 'Pornography and Censorship', in Michael S Kimmel (ed.), *Men Confront Pornography*, Meridian, New York, 1990.

'Testosterone and Androgens in Women', Women's Health Program, Monash University, 15 March 2005, http://womenshealth.med.monash.edu.au/documents/testosterone-in-women.pdf, viewed September 2008.

Tiefer, Leonore, *Sex Is Not a Natural Act and Other Essays*, Westview Press, Boulder, CO, 1995.

'Tom', 'Getting Back in the Game: Impotency, PCa and the Single Man', Phoenix 5, March 2000, www.phoenix5.org/stories/firstpers/perstomimpot.html, viewed November 2008.

Tsing Loh, Sandra, 'She's Just Not That into You', *Atlantic Monthly*, March 2007, www.theatlantic.com/doc/200703/loh-libido, viewed September 2008.

Urban, Rebecca, 'Rough Ride to Smooth Wrinkles', *Age*, 22 May 2004.

'Voice of Australian Women', *Australian Women's Weekly*, April 2008.

Weiner Davis, Michele, *The Sex-starved Marriage*, Simon and Schuster, London, 2003.

——*The Sex-starved Wife: What to Do When He's Lost Desire*, Simon and Schuster, New York, 2008.

Widmer, Eric R, Judith Treas and Robert Newcomb, 'Attitudes Towards Non-marital Sex in 24 Countries', *Journal of Sex Research*, November 1998, pp. 349–58.

Wolcott, Ilene and Jody Hughes, 'Towards Understanding the Reasons for Divorce', working paper no. 20, AIFS, Melbourne, June 1999.

Zilbergeld, Bernie, *The New Male Sexuality: The Truth about Men, Sex and Pleasure*, Bantam, New York, 1992.

Index